EMQs for the

EMQs for the MRCOG Part 2

Mirka Slavska, MD, DFSRH, MRCOG
Senior Registrar in obstetrics and gynaecology
University Hospital of Wales, Cardiff

Charity J. Knight, MBChB, MRCOG, BSc (Hons), DFSRH, PgCert MedEd (Merit)
Consultant obstetrician and gynaecologist
Singleton Hospital, Swansea

EMQs for the MRCOG Part 2

Published by:
Anshan Ltd
6 Newlands Road
Tunbridge Wells
Kent. TN4 9AT

Tel: +44 (0) 1892 557767
Fax: +44 (0) 1892 530358

e-mail: info@anshan.co.uk
website: www.anshan.co.uk

© 2019 Anshan Ltd

ISBN: 9781848291447

All rights reserved. No part of this publication may be reproduced, stored in a retrieval system, or transmitted in any form or by any means, electronic, mechanical, photocopying, recording or otherwise, without the prior written permission of the publisher.

The use of registered names, trademarks, etc, in this publication does not imply, even in the absence of a specific statement that such names are exempt from the relevant laws and regulations and therefore for general use.

While every effort has been made to ensure the accuracy of the information contained within this publication, the publisher can give no guarantee for information about drug dosage and application thereof contained in this book. In every individual case the respective user must check current indications and accuracy by consulting other pharmaceutical literature and following the guidelines laid down by the manufacturers of specific products and the relevant authorities in the country in which they are practicing.

British Library Cataloguing in Publication Data

A catalogue record for this book is available from the British Library.

Every effort has been made to trace all copyright holders, but if any have been inadvertently overlooked the publishers will be pleased to make the necessary arrangements at the first opportunity.

Copy Editor: Andrew White
Cover and Image Design: Emma Randall

Typeset by: Kerrypress Ltd, St Albans, Hertfordshire
Printed and bound by: GraphyCems Spain

Introduction

Preface

Spurred on by the success of our first publication 'SBAs for the MRCOG Part 2,' we decided to undertake a second challenge- 'EMQs for the MRCOG Part 2.' We realised that there were few up to date EMQ revision books covering the most recent guidelines that had been published. We had both been obstetric and gynaecology registrars who had completed the MRCOG whilst in training in the United Kingdom, so we recognized the need to have current material, provided in a simple format, with references available to maximize study time.

We have divided this book into an obstetric section and a gynaecology section, with each containing two complete exam papers. You can use these questions either throughout your revision preparation or as mock papers to fully prepare yourself prior to the exam day.

We hope that this up to date EMQ exam preparation book will assist your learning in the great challenge of successfully passing the "Part 2" and wish you the very best of luck.

Format of the MRCOG Part 2 Exam

The MRCOG Part 2 examination is the second written component of the membership exam. The exam is conducted over one day and is composed of two papers. Each paper lasts 3 hours, with a much needed one hour break in between. Each paper has equal marks and is composed of 50 Extended Matching Questions (EMQs) (worth 60% of the marks) and 50 Single Best Answer (SBAs) questions (worth 40% of the marks.) The RCOG recommends spending 110 minutes on the EMQs and 70 minutes on the SBA questions. Only with successful completion of the Part 2 exam can you proceed to the Part 3 exam, which is an oral examination (OSCE) that once successfully completed, will lead to you being awarded the MRCOG. (RCOG, 2018.)

At the start of each exam you will be handed an EMQ question booklet and an EMQ answer sheet. Each tranche of questions contains an option list presented in a table format, (each option is lettered and in alphabetical or numerical order,) followed by an introductory statement then between one and five questions. The corresponding answer sheet is laid out with answers from 1-50, with each answer containing 20 boxes (which the College calls "lozenges") that are labelled A-T. The option list will not use all of these boxes, usually giving between ten and fourteen answer options. You need to select the answer of your choice by shading-in the appropriate box with the pencil provided. There is not a negative marking scheme, so always try to answer every question. However if more than one answer has been filled in, then no marks will be given (even if one of the answers is correct,) so try to erase any errors completely. (RCOG, 2018.)

What is an EMQ?

EMQ stands for Extended Matching Questions, which is a form of multiple choice questioning. They have been successfully used in the MRCOG Part 2 exam since 2006. The EMQ aims to test not only factual recall but also to elicit a greater understanding of the theory, and apply it to a clinical setting. The questions have also been found to examine clinical problem-solving effectively, with well maintained reliability. (Duthie et al, 2006.) The Part 2 EMQ format means that there are between ten and fourteen potential options which can be selected as the correct answer, thus making it exceedingly difficult to guess the correct option.

How should I prepare for the exam?

It is really important that you give yourself adequate time to fully prepare for the exam and we suggest at least six months prior to the January or July exam dates. Your reference sources should include all of the RCOG guidelines: Green Top Guidelines; Good Practice Guidelines, Scientific Impact Papers; patient information leaflets and TOG articles, as well as NICE Guidelines, SIGN Guidelines and StratOG modules. Use of exam preparation books like this one will give you a good idea of the exam format.

Attending an MRCOG written exam preparation course can also give you a more in-depth exposure to topics which may come up in the exam, often with lots of EMQ and SBA example questions provided. Many courses will also provide you with a mock examination to give you a more realistic examination experience prior to the real event.

References

RCOG, 2018. (www.rcog.org.uk)

Duthie S, Hodges P, Ramsay I, Reid W. EMQs: A new component of the MRCOG Part 2 exam.TOG, 2006; 8: 181-185.

ABBREVIATIONS

ACS	Acute chest syndrome
AFI	Amniotic fluid index
AFP	Alpha-fetoprotein
ALSG	Advanced life support group
ALT	Alanine aminotransferase
ANC	Antenatal clinic
APTT	Activated partial thromboplastin time test
BA	Bile acids
BD	Bis die – twice daily
bHCG	Beta human chorionic gonadotropin
BMI	Body mass index
BPS	Bladder pain syndrome
BSE	Bovine spongiform encephalopathy
CA125	Cancer antigen 125
CABG	Coronary artery bypass graft
CBT	Cognitive behavioural therapy
cffDNA	Cell-free foetal DNA
cfu	Colony-forming unit
CHC	Combined hormonal contraceptive
CIN-3	Cervical intra-epithelial neoplasia 3
CMV	Cytomegalovirus
Coag	Coagulation screen
COCP	Combined oral contraceptive pill
COPD	Chronic obstructive pulmonary disease
C/S or C-section	Caesarean section
CSP	Cervical screening programming
CT	Computed tomography
CTG	Cardiotocography
Cu-IUD	Copper intrauterine device
DCDA	Dichorionic diamniotic
DES	Diethylstilbestrol
DEXA/DXA	Dual energy X-ray absorptiometry

DNA	Deoxyribonucleic acid
DVT	Deep vein thrombosis
dw	Dry weight
EAS muscle	External anal sphincter muscle
EBV	Epstein-Barr virus
ECV	External cephalic version
EC	Emergency contraception
ECHO	Echocardiogram
FBC	Full blood count
FBS	Foetal blood sampling
FFP	Fresh frozen plasma
FMH	Fetomaternal haemorrhage
FSH	Follicle-stimulating hormone
GBS	Group B streptococcus
GnRH analogue	Gonadotrophin releasing hormone
GP	General practitioner
GUM	Genito-urinary medicine
Hb	Haemoglobin
hCG	Human chorionic gonadotropin
HDFN/HDN	Haemolytic disease of the foetus and neonate
HELLP	Haemolysis, elevated LFTs, low platelets
HMB	Heavy menstrual bleeding
HPV	Human papilloma virus
HR	High risk
HRT	Hormone replacement therapy
HSIL	High grade squamous intraepithelial lesion (also known as VIN2/3)
IAP	Intrapartum antibiotic prophylaxis
IAS muscle	Internal anal sphincter muscle
IBD	Inflammatory bowel disease
ICD	International classification of diseases
IM	Intramuscular
IMP	Implant
IOL	Induction of labour
IR	Immediate release
ITP	Idiopathic thrombocytopaenic purpura
ITU	Intensive treatment unit
IU	In utero
IUC/IUCD/IUD	Intra-uterine contraceptive device

IUS	Intra-uterine system
IUT	Intra-uterine transfusion
i.v.	Intravenous
IVDU	Intravenous drug user
IVF	In vitro fertilisation
LDH	Lactate dehydrogenase
LFTs	Liver function tests
LH	Luteinizing hormone
LLETZ	Large loop excision of the transformation zone
LMWH	Low molecular weight heparin
LNG-EC	Levonorgestrel emergency contraception
LNG-IUS	Levonorgestrel intra-uterine system
LSIL	Low grade squamous intraepithelial lesion (also known as VIN1)
MBL	Measured blood loss
MCA PSV	Middle cerebral artery peak systolic velocity
MDT	Multi-disciplinary team
MM	Maternal mortality
MOET	Managing obstetric emergencies and trauma
MoM	Multiples of the median
MOH	Major obstetric haemorrhage
MRI	Magnetic resonance imaging
MRKH	Mayer-Rokitansky-Kuster-Hauser Syndrome
MSU	Midstream specimen of urine
NSAID	Non-steroidal anti-inflammatory drug
OAB	Over-active bladder
Od	Once daily
OHSS	Ovarian hyperstimulation syndrome
OP	Outpatient
PCOS	Polycystic ovary syndrome
PDS	Polydioxynone suture
PE	Pulmonary embolism
PET	Pre-eclamptic toxaemia
PID	Pelvic inflammatory disease
PLT	Platelets
PMH	Past medical history
PMS	Pre-menstrual syndrome
p.o.	Per os - orally
PN	Postnatal

POI	Premature ovarian insufficiency
POP	Progestorone-only pill
P-PROM	Preterm-prelabour rupture of membranes
PT	Prothrombin time test
PTNS	Percutaneous tibial nerve stimulation
RAADP	Routine antenatal anti-D Ig prophylaxis
RBC	Red blood cells
RHD	Rhesus D
RTA	Road traffic accident
rVIIa	Recombinant factor VIIa
s.c.	Sub cutaneous
SCD	Sickle cell disease
SOB	Shortness of breath
SROM	Spontaneous rupture of membranes
SSRI	Serotonin specific reuptake inhibitor
STEMI	ST-elevation myocardial infarction
SVD	Spontaneous vaginal delivery
TPO	Thyroid peroxidase
TXA	Tranexamic acid
UAE	Uterine artery embolisation
UE	Urea and electrolytes
UI	Urinary incontinence
UKMEC	United Kingdom medical eligibility criteria
UPA-EC	Ulipristal acetate emergency contraceptive
UPSI	Unprotected sexual intercourse
USS	Ultrasound scan
UTI	Urinary tract infection
WHO	World Health Organisation
VTE	Venous thromboembolism
21-OH	21-Hydroxylase

TABLE OF CONTENTS

Introduction   i
Abbreviations   v

QUESTIONS

Gynaecology paper 1 – Questions   1
Obstetrics paper 1 – Questions   23
Gynaecology paper 2 – Questions   45
Obstetrics paper 2 – Questions   69

ANSWERS

Gynaecology paper 1 – Answers   93
Obstetrics paper 1 – Answers   105
Gynaecology paper 2 – Answers   123
Obstetrics paper 2 – Answers   137

Gynaecology paper 1 - Questions

Options for questions 1 - 2

    A. Cyclical use of drospirenone-containing COC

    B. Continuous use of drospirenone-containing COC

    C. Percutaneous estradiol and progestogen

    D. Micronised progesterone

    E. Danazol 200 mg BD

    F. GnRH analogues

    G. GnRH analogue and tibolone

    H. Progesterone

    I. LNG-IUS

    J. Spironolactone

    K. Hysterectomy and bilateral salpingo-oophorectomy

    L. Hysterectomy with conservation of ovaries

    M. Vitex agnus castus

    N. Fluoxetine in luteal phase

    O. SSRI in luteal phase

    P. Endometrial ablation

Instructions

For each clinical scenario below, choose the single most appropriate management option from the list. Each option maybe used once, more than once, or not at all.

1. A 28-year-old lady has been referred by her GP with a lack of concentration, mood swings, irritability, breast tenderness, bloating and food cravings two weeks before her period starts. She has seen a counsellor and her symptoms improved for a few months but now they have returned. She is fit and well. Her partner is in the navy and they are not planning to start a family yet. What would be the best treatment option for her?

2. A 32-year-old lady with a BMI of 29 has been referred by her GP with severe PMS symptoms. She has been throwing plates at her husband before she gets her period. She has two children delivered vaginally and her family is now complete. She had a DVT four years ago following a knee operation. Her periods are heavy. What would be the best treatment option for her?

Options for questions 3 - 6

A. Kelly plication

B. Marshall-Marchetti-Krantz procedure

C. Paravaginal deficit repair

D. Urodynamics

E. Refer to tertiary centre

F. MDT

G. Botox A

H. Percutaneous sacral nerve stimulation

I. Autologous rectus fascial sling

J. Duloxetine

K. Desmopressin

L. Oxybutynin

M. Mirabegron

N. Tolterodine

O. Darifenacin

P. Oestrogen cream vaginally

Q. Percutaneous posterior tibial nerve stimulation

R. Pad test

Instructions

For each clinical scenario below, choose the single most likely management option from the list. Each option maybe used once, more than once, or not at all.

3. A 77-year-old lady with a BMI of 23 presents with frequency of urination, urgency and nocturia with 4 episodes per night. She drinks 2 cups of decaffeinated tea per day and has been told by her GP not to drink after 19:00. She is on multiple medications. On examination you find that she has no prolapse, pelvic floor muscle tone has an Oxford Scale 4 and the vagina appears atrophic.

4. A 90-year-old lady complains that she needs to pass water too often during the day and whenever she feels the sensation to urinate she has to find a toilet very quickly, otherwise she would have an accident. She gets up 4 times during the night and complains that she is tired all the time. She has a normal BMI and is taking thyroxine. Examination reveals a postmenopausal vulva and vagina with no cervical descent or vaginal wall prolapse.

5. A 32-year-old mother of twins delivered vaginally 4 years ago presented with leaking on coughing and when she runs. She is fit and healthy with no evidence of vaginal prolapse. You referred her to physiotherapy, which had some benefit, but she is not completely happy with the result. She isn't sure that her family is complete.

6. A 58-year-old lady who regularly plays golf with her friends is troubled with leaking when she coughs or laughs. She also has the need to pass water almost every hour, and if she can't find a toilet she will have an accident. She gets up 3 times in the night to pass urine. Your colleague has referred her for bladder training which has not worked well, and hence she was commenced on oxybutinin. You review her in clinic 3 months later with little improvement in symptoms and an intolerable dry mouth. What would you do next?

Options for questions 7 - 9

A. Ultrasound scan

B. Discharge from follow up

C. Laparoscopy

D. Laparoscopy and oophorectomy

E. Laparoscopy and de-torsion of the ovary

F. Laparotomy

G. Oophoropexy

H. Consider MRI

I. Consider CT

J. CA 125

K. CA 125, LDH

L. CA 125, LDH, bHCG, AFP

Instructions

For each clinical scenario below, choose the single most important management option from the list. Each option maybe used once, more than once, or not at all.

7. A 14-year-old girl with a normal BMI and regular periods presents to A&E with left iliac fossa pain and vomiting. She is not sexually active. Her last period was 3 weeks ago. A pelvic ultrasound scan reported an enlarged and hyperechoic left ovary with peripherally displaced follicles and hyperechoic stroma. There is little intra-ovarian venous flow on assessment with Doppler. Some free fluid in Pouch of Douglas.

8. A 13-year-old girl who achieved menarche a few months ago has a pelvic ultrasound scan which describes a simple ovarian cyst of the right ovary measuring 4.6 cm size. There are no other features reported on the scan.

9. A 14-year-old girl who has been having regular menstrual periods for the last 2 years has had an incidental finding of a simple right sided ovarian cyst measuring 6.8 cm. She has no symptoms.

Options for questions 10 - 12

　　A. 2-5:1000 procedures in 10 years

　　B. Up to 15% of bowel injuries might not be diagnosed at the time of surgery

　　C. 1 in 10

　　D. 1 in 20

　　E. 4 in 100

　　F. 9 in 100

　　G. 11 in 100

　　H. 21 in 100

　　I. 3-6 in 1000

　　J. 1 in 2000

　　K. None of the above

Instructions

For each procedure below, choose the single most appropriate option from the list. Each option maybe used once, more than once, or not at all.

10. Risk of bowel injury at diagnostic laparoscopy

11. The overall risk of serious complications from abdominal hysterectomy

12. Lifetime failure rate for laparoscopic tubal occlusion with clips

Options for questions 13 - 15

A. Complete androgen sensitivity syndrome
B. Congenital adrenal hyperplasia
C. Fragile X syndrome
D. Imperforate hymen
E. Klinefelter syndrome
F. Kallmann syndrome
G. McCune-Albright syndrome
H. Mayer Rokitansky Küster Hauser syndrome (MRKH)
I. Partial androgen insensitivity syndrome
J. Swyer syndrome
K. Transverse lower vaginal septum
L. Turner's syndrome

Instructions

For each clinical scenario below, choose the single most likely diagnosis. Each option maybe used once, more than once, or not at all.

13. A 15-year-old girl presents with primary amenorrhoea and dyspareunia. She has normal secondary sexual characteristics. A pelvic ultrasound scan reports an aplastic uterus with small ovaries. Her karyotype is 46,XX. On examination you see a short blind-ending vagina.

14. A 17-year-old girl presents with primary amenorrhoea and dyspareunia. She has developed breasts but no axillary or pubic hair. Her karyotype is 46,XY. On examination you see a short blind-ending vagina.

15. A 16-year-old girl presents with delayed onset of puberty. She has primary amenorrhoea, normal genitalia and no breast development, but she has some sparse axillary and pubic hair. Pelvic ultrasound revealed a small uterus and ovaries were not seen. Karyotype is 46,XY.

Options for questions 16 - 20

A. Avoid intercourse

B. Copper coil

C. Too late for emergency contraception

D. Defer oral contraceptive for 5 days

E. Defer oral contraceptive for 7 days

F. Oestrogen

G. LNG oral emergency contraceptive

H. LNG oral emergency contraceptive double dose 3 mg

I. Mirena coil

J. Perform pregnancy test

K. Start oral contraceptive pill

L. UPA oral emergency contraceptive

M. UPA oral emergency contraceptive double dose

Instructions

For each statement below, select the single most appropriate management option from the list. Each option maybe used once, more than once, or not at all.

16. Most effective method of emergency contraception.

17. EC effective up to 120 hours after UPSI.

18. EC licenced up to 72 hours after UPSI.

19. EC ineffective if taken 96 hours after UPSI.

20. The effectiveness of this contraceptive method is not affected by weight or BMI.

Options for questions 21 - 23

A. 1
B. 2
C. 3
D. 4
E. 5
F. 6
G. 8
H. 9
I. 10
J. 12
K. 15
L. 20
M. 24
N. 25

Instructions

For each clinical scenario below, choose the single most appropriate option from the list. Each option maybe used once, more than once, or not at all.

21. A 68-year-old lady presented to gynaecology clinic with post-menopausal bleeding. You obtained an endometrial biopsy and the histology reports endometrial hyperplasia without atypia. How will you counsel her when she asks you what percentage of cases will progress to endometrial cancer?

22. A 76-year-old lady presented to gynaecology clinic with post-menopausal bleeding. You obtained an endometrial biopsy and the histology reports endometrial hyperplasia without atypia. She agrees to take norethisterone and asks how long she will have to take the treatment for. What is the minimum duration of treatment (in months)?

23. A 70-year-old lady presented to gynaecology clinic with post-menopausal bleeding. You obtained an endometrial biopsy and the histology reports endometrial hyperplasia without atypia. She agrees to take norethisterone but there is no sign of histological regression on repeat biopsy. She asks you how long she should continue the progestogen treatment for before considering a hysterectomy?

Options for questions 24 -25

A. Bowen's disease of the vulva
B. Herpes simplex infection
C. HSIL of vulva
D. Human papillomavirus infection
E. Lichen planus
F. Lichen sclerosus
G. Lichen simplex
H. LSIL of vulva
I. Vulval candidiasis
J. Vulval eczema
K. Vulval intraepithelial neoplasia
L. Vulval psoriasis
M Provoked vulvodynia
N. Unprovoked vulvodynia

Instructions

For each clinical scenario below, choose the single most likely diagnosis/appropriate treatment option from the list. Each option maybe used once, more than once, or not at all.

24. A 64-year-old lady presents to gynaecology clinic with vulval itch and general soreness. She has had recurrent UTIs in the past year and describes superficial dyspareunia. She has tried hydrocortisone cream but this hasn't helped much. She has a past medical history of hypothyroidism. On examination the vulva appears atrophic with labial fusion, burying of the clitoris and narrowing of the introitus with fissures evident.

25. A 48-year-old lady presents to gynaecology clinic with a history of vulval itch and soreness, describing a burning sensation which was worse at nights. She has no relevant past medical history, but on further questioning says she has noticed red itchy lesions in the axillae. On examination there are well demarcated, symmetrical, erythematous plaques affecting the labia majora, groins and natal cleft, with grey scaly patches extending down the inner thighs.

Options for questions 26 - 28

A. Lifestyle advice

B. Vaginal oestrogen pessary

C. Vaginal oestrogen ring

D. Oestrogen implant

E. Continuous combined HRT

F. Sequential HRT

G. Topical oestrogen

H. Oestrogen and progesterone patch

I. Topical oestrogen and Mirena IUS

J. Testosterone gel

K. Testosterone implant

L. Fluoxetine

M. Black cohosh

N. St John's Wort

O. Cognitive behavioural therapy

Instructions

For each clinical scenario below, choose the single most appropriate management option from the list. Each option maybe used once, more than once, or not at all.

26. A 56-year-old lady went through the menopause 3 years ago. She has a new partner and is bothered by vaginal dryness and pain during sexual intercourse.

27. A 54-year-old lady went through the menopause 2 years ago. She has terrible hot flushes and wakes every hour with night sweats. She is exhausted and wants hormonal treatment. She developed a DVT following a knee operation two years ago. What treatment would you recommend?

28. A 51-year-old lady went through the menopause 4 years ago. She has terrible hot flushes and night sweats. She has difficulty concentrating and feels low in mood. She wants hormonal treatment. She developed a DVT following a total hysterectomy procedure for fibroids when she was 40. What treatment would you recommend?

Options for questions 29 - 31

A. Clomiphene citrate
B. Eflornithine (topical)
C. Gonadotrophin therapy
D. Laparoscopic ovarian diathermy
E. Letrozole
F. Lifestyle changes
G. Metformin
H. Mirena IUS
I. Norethisterone (cyclical)
J. Novorapid
K. Simvastatin
L. Spironolactone
M. Yasmin
N. None of the above

Instructions

For each clinical scenario below, choose the single most appropriate treatment option from the list. Each option maybe used once, more than once, or not at all.

29. A 21-year-old lady with PCOS presents with troublesome hirsutism. She has a BMI of 47. She had little effect from 9 months of topical eflornithine prescribed by the GP.

30. A 19-year-old lady with PCOS presented to clinic with hirsutism. She tried topical eflornithine with little effect. She has a BMI of 25. She does not want to start a family at present.

31. A 27-year-old lady with PCOS has been amenorrhoeic for 2 years. She has a BMI of 48. She declined oral treatment because she struggles to swallow tablets.

Options for questions 32 - 33

A. Appendicitis
B. Bladder pain syndrome
C. Diverticulitis
D. Ectopic pregnancy
E. Endometriosis
F. Ovarian cyst torsion
G. Over active bladder
H. Pelvic congestion syndrome
I. Pelvic inflammatory disease
J. Renal stone
K. Ruptured ovarian cyst
L. Urodynamic stress incontinence
M. Urinary tract infection
N. None of the above

Instructions

For each clinical scenario below, choose the single most likely diagnosis from the list. Each option maybe used once, more than once, or not at all.

32. A 34-year-old lady presented with a 2 year history of central pelvic pain, pressure, persistent urinary frequency and urgency. Urine dipstick was negative and microscopy and culture had never grown any infections. Renal and pelvic ultrasound scans were normal. A trial of oxybutynin, darifenacin then mirabegron proved ineffective. Urodynamic studies were entirely normal. A cystoscopy reported post-distension glomerulations.

33. A 48-year-old lady presented to gynaecology clinic with symptoms of prolapse. She is a Para 2 (she had a forceps delivery and a normal vaginal delivery.) She also reports urinary incontinence after coughing, dysuria, urinary frequency and urgency. MSU was negative.

Options for questions 34 - 35

A. Check karyotype

B. Perform test for Fragile X permutation

C. Check for 21-OH antibodies and TPO antibodies

D. Perform diabetes screening

E. Perform infection screening

F. Refer to cardiologist, geneticist and endocrinologist

G. Book for gonadectomy

H. Commence POP

I. Arrange DEXA scan annually

J. Arrange DEXA scan 5 yearly

Instructions

For each clinical scenario below, choose the single most appropriate management option from the list. Each option maybe used once, more than once, or not at all.

34. A 23-year-old lady presents with primary amenorrhoea and FSH level of 48 which was done by her GP. She returns for a follow up appointment in gynaecology clinic when you tell her that the results of karyotyping show XY chromosomes.

35. A 38-year-old lady presents with amenorrhoea for 14 months and FSH level of 36. She is fit and well but is a known asthmatic, suffers with hay fever and you note atopic dermatitis on her forearms. She's never had any surgery. She has one healthy child and no significant family history.

Options for questions 36 - 40

A. Abdominal hysterectomy
B. COCP
C. GnRH analogue
D. Jaydess IUS
E. POP
F. Lifestyle advice
G. LNG IUS
H. Norethisterone
I. Tranexamic acid
J. Mefenamic acid
K. Endometrial ablation
L. Supra-cervical laparoscopic hysterectomy
M. Uterine artery embolisation
N. Vaginal hysterectomy
O. Yasmin
P. None of the above

Instructions

Select the most appropriate treatment for each clinical case outlined below.

36. A 24-year-old lady presented with menorrhagia. She had a BMI of 29 and also complained of hirsutism. She was sexually active, using condoms for contraception.

37. A 42-year-old lady presented to clinic with menorrhagia and recurrent CIN 3. She was a Para 2 having 2 normal deliveries. She had previously tried hormonal contraceptives including LNG IUS with little effect. She underwent endometrial ablation two years ago but her symptoms have worsened. On examination she has stage 1 uterine descent.

38. A 45-year-old lady presents to gynaecology clinic with longstanding menorrhagia. She is a Para 3 (3 vaginal deliveries.) She has previously tried tranexamic acid and had endometrial ablation 4 years ago but her symptoms have worsened. She has a PMH of breast cancer and has just commenced tamoxifen.

39. A 39-year-old lady presents to gynaecology clinic with worsening menorrhagia. A pelvic ultrasound reports an enlarged uterus containing numerous fibroids, with the largest measuring 10cm x 9cm. She has tried hormonal treatments including a Mirena IUS and hysteroscopic myomectomy with little benefit.

40. A 44-year-old lady presents to gynaecology clinic with worsening menorrhagia. She has a PMH of breast cancer. She declines any hormonal treatment or operative intervention.

Options for questions 41 - 43

A. Amitriptyline
B. Cimetidine
C. Desmopressin
D. Duloxetine
L. Gabapentin
N. Intravesical bacillus Calmette-Guerin
G. Intravesical lidocaine
H. Intravesical resiniferatoxin
I. Mirabegron
J. Oxybutynin IR
K. Posterior tibial nerve stimulation
M. Sacral neuromodulation
N. Tolterodine
O. None of the above

Instructions

For each clinical scenario below, choose the most appropriate treatment option from the list. Each option maybe used once, more than once, or not at all.

41. A 42-year-old lady has been diagnosed with bladder pain syndrome. She has tried conservative and oral treatments which haven't been effective.

42. A 30-year-old lady has been diagnosed with bladder pain syndrome. She has tried co-codamol and ibuprofen which haven't helped.

43. A 48-year-old lady has been diagnosed with bladder pain syndrome. She has tried conservative, pharmacological and intravesical treatments but nothing has proved effective. She is keen to avoid any operative procedures.

Options for questions 44 – 48

- A. Colposcopy
- B. Colposcopy + biopsy
- C. Cease recall for age reasons
- D. Colposcopy, see and treat
- E. Cytology at 6 months
- F. Gynaecology referral
- G. HPV test
- H. MDT
- I. Routine recall
- J. Hysterectomy
- K. LLETZ
- L. Cone biopsy
- M. High vaginal swab
- N. No need for cervical smear

Gynaecology paper 1 – Questions

Instructions

For each clinical scenario below, choose the single most appropriate management option from the list. Each option maybe used once, more than once, or not at all.

44. A 48-year-old lady has undergone a routine smear. It showed that there was low grade dyskariosis.

45. A 44-year-old woman with a BMI of 41 had abnormal endometrial cells on her smear sample.

46. Normal endometrial cells were reported on a 41-year-old woman's smear result.

47. A 34-year-old lady had a third, consecutive cervical smear result reported as inadequate.

48. A 27-year-old lady who had a normal smear two years ago but is a heavy smoker is commenced on an oral contraceptive by her GP.

Options for questions 49 – 50

A. No need for anti-D

B. Give 250 IU anti-D

C. Give 250 IU anti-D and request Kleihauer

D. Discuss with haematology lab how much extra anti-D is needed

E. Give 500 IU anti-D

F. Give 500 IU anti-D and request Kleihauer

G. Give 500 IU anti-D and request Kleihauer, both within 72 hours from delivery

H. Give 500 IU anti-D and request Kleihauer, both within 72 hours from diagnosis of IUD

I. Give 1500 IU anti-D

J. Request cffDNA

K. None of the above

Instructions

For each clinical scenario below, choose the single most appropriate management option from the list. Each option maybe used once, more than once, or not at all.

49. A 19-year-old G1P0 Rhesus negative lady who was at 9 weeks gestation had a complete miscarriage. She had moderate vaginal bleeding and minimal pain.

50. A 28-year-old G4P2 Rhesus negative non-sensitised lady underwent medical management of an ectopic pregnancy at 7 weeks gestation.

Obstetrics paper 1 - Questions

Options for questions 1 - 3

A. No admission, no treatment, BP once a week, urinary protein analysis once a week.

B. No admission, no treatment, BP once a week, urinary protein analysis once a week, PET bloods.

C. No admission, no treatment, BP 2X per week, urinary protein analysis 2X per week.

D. No admission, treat until BP <140/90, BP 2X per week, urinary protein analysis 2X per week.

E. No admission, treat until BP <150/100, BP 2X per week, urinary protein analysis 2X per week.

F. No admission, treat until BP <150/100, BP 2X per week, urinary protein analysis 2X per week, PET bloods.

G. Admit, treat until BP < 140/90, BP once a day, urinary protein analysis once a week.

H. Admit, treat until BP < 150/100, BP once a day, urinary protein analysis once a week.

I. Admit, treat until BP < 150/100, BP once a day, urinary protein analysis once a week, PET bloods.

J. Admit, treat until BP <140/90, BP 4X daily, urinary protein analysis daily, PET bloods.

K. Admit, treat until BP <150/100, BP 4X daily, urinary protein analysis daily, PET bloods.

Instructions

For each clinical scenario, select the most appropriate management option from the list above. Each option maybe used once, more than once, or not at all.

1. A 21-year-old G1P0 with BMI of 32 and blood pressure measuring 145/95 mmHg, no proteinuria at 26 weeks gestation, is currently on no anti-hypertensive treatment.

2. A 25-year-old G1P0 with BMI of 32 and blood pressure measuring 145/95 mmHg, no proteinuria at 35 weeks gestation, is currently on no anti-hypertensive treatment.

3. A 31-year-old G1P0 with BMI of 38 and blood pressure measuring 145/95 at 35 weeks gestation has no proteinuria and takes no anti-hypertensive medication.

Options for questions 4 - 6

A. Start ursodeoxycholic acid + Piriton + vitamin K

B. Start ursodeoxycholic acid + Piriton

C. Start cholestyramine

D. Prescribe vitamin K 5-10 mg daily

E. Repeat LFTs in 1-2 weeks

F. Repeat LFTs, UE, FBC, Coag, BA in 1-2 weeks

G. Refer to gastroenterologist

H. Arrange USS for foetal growth + AFI

I. Give steroids

J. Perform hepatitis A, hepatitis B, hepatitis C, EBV, CMV, anti-smooth muscle antibodies, anti-mitochondrial antibodies tests and USS liver

K. Start S-Adenosyl methionine (SAMe)

L. Deliver

M. Wait and see

Instructions

Select the most appropriate next step in the management of the cases described below. Each option maybe used once, more than once, or not at all.

4. A 21-year-old G2P1 (SVDX1) at 23 weeks gestation presents to the obstetric assessment unit with constant itch of the palms and soles of her feet, which gets worse in the night. Investigations are normal but she is still itchy. What's the next step?

5. The same woman has slightly increased BA, ALT 18 IU/L, normal coagulation screen and normal FBC at 28 weeks. She continues to be itchy. What would you do?

6. The same woman is found to have a PT of 21 seconds (prolonged) at 35 weeks. What would you do?

Options for questions 7 - 8

A. Manage in community with regular analgesia

B. Give analgesia within 30 minutes of arrival and give effective analgesia in 1 hour

C. Exchange transfusion

D. Top up transfusion

E. Discuss delivery after 38 weeks

F. Admit

G. Consider admission to critical care unit and therapeutic thromboprophylaxis

H. Prophylactic thromboprophylaxis

I. Thrombolysis

J. MRI

K. Broad spectrum antibiotics

L. Give steroid

M. Observe

Instructions

For each clinical scenario below, choose the most appropriate management option from the list. Each option maybe used once, more than once, or not at all.

7. A 23-year-old lady who is G1P0 at 21+3 weeks gestation with sickle cell disease is on penicillin prophylaxis. She presents with pain in her hips, elbows, left upper quadrant (per abdomen) and headache. She is feeling nauseous but hasn't vomited. Her temperature is 37.10C. She was given paracetamol and ibuprofen in A&E with good effect. Her haemoglobin is 7.1 g/l, UE and LFTs are normal. CXR is clear.

8. A 21-year-old woman who is G2P1 at 24+2 weeks gestation is known to have SCD. She has been taking aspirin since 12 weeks. She presents with left sided weakness, slurred speech and tunnel vision which started 1 hour ago and is not resolving.

Options for questions 9 - 11

A. Monitor 4 weekly up to 24 weeks then 2 weekly until delivery
B. Monitor 4 weekly up to 28 weeks then 2 weekly until delivery
C. Refer to foetal medicine for IUT
D. Refer to foetal medicine
E. Monitor by MCA PSV every 2 weeks
F. Monitor by MCA PSV every week
G. Deliver
H. Request cffDNA for foetal genotype at 12 weeks
I. Request cffDNA for foetal genotype at 16 weeks
J. Request cffDNA for foetal genotype at 20 weeks
K. Observe
L. Amniocentesis in 5 weeks time
M. Amniocentesis in 12 weeks time

Instructions

For each clinical scenario below, choose the single most appropriate management option from the list. Each option maybe used once, more than once, or not at all.

9. A G2P1 who is 16 weeks pregnant has got an Anti-D titre of 2.5.

10. A G2P1 who is 12 weeks gestation has got Anti-E and Anti-c titres of 1.3 (slightly above normal.)

11. A G2P1 who is 29 weeks pregnant has got an Anti-K titre of 3.8.

Options for questions 12 - 13

A. Cryoprecipitate, two 5 unit pools to be given early in MOH and then depending on fibrinogen levels

B. Cryoprecipitate, one 5 unit pool to be given early in MOH and then depending on fibrinogen levels

C. 12 units RBC, cryoprecipitate, FFP 12-15 ml/kg for every 6 units RBC then depending on clotting and anti-D

D. 12 units RBC, cryoprecipitate, FFP 12-15 ml/kg for every 6 units RBC then depending on clotting and platelets

E. 12 units RBC, cryoprecipitate, FFP 12-15 ml/kg for every 6 units RBC then depending on clotting

F. Anti-D

G. FFP 12-15 ml/kg for every 6 units RBC then depending on clotting

H. 2 units Rh negative platelets to be given through platelets giving set and 250 i.u. anti-D

I. 2 units Rh positive platelets to be given through platelets giving set and 250 i.u. anti-D

J. 2 units Rh negative platelets to be given through platelets giving set

K. Tranexamic acid

L. rVIIa

M. Fibrinogen concentrate

N. Decide on clinical and haematological grounds

O. Give 0 RhD negative blood

P. None of the above

Instructions

For each clinical scenario below, choose the single most appropriate management option from the list. Each option maybe used once, more than once, or not at all.

12. A 27-year-old para 3 had a vaginal delivery 2 hours ago. She is Rh D negative and is now bleeding heavily with a current MBL of 4.8 L. She has already received 9 units of red blood cells and FFP. Her haemoglobin on HemoCue is 62 g/l, platelets 106, fibrinogen 1.3 g/l

13. A 39-year-old Rh negative, A blood group lady who is known to have ITP has just had an emergency C-section. Blood results just back show: Hb is 90 g/l, platelets 48 X109/l, fibrinogen 3.1 g/l, PT and APTT are normal. She is bleeding moderately during the procedure.

Options for questions 14 - 16

    A. Low dose aspirin

    B. Low dose aspirin and LMWH prophylaxis

    C. Thromboprophylaxis

    D. Folic acid 5 g

    E. Folic acid 400 mg

    F. Transfuse 2-3 units RBC until Hb 100 g/l, then top up in a week until Hb 120-130 g/l

    G. Aim for top up of 2 RBC units at 37-38 weeks

    H. Aim for top up of 2 RBC units at 39-40 weeks

    I. Chelation therapy p.o.

    J. Chelation therapy i.v.

    K. Chelation therapy s.c.

    L. Desferrioxamine 2g/24 hrs i.v

    M. Liver MRI

    N. Refer to surgeons

    O. USS for viability

    P. Wait and see

Instructions

For each clinical scenario below, choose the single most appropriate management option from the list. Each option maybe used once, more than once, or not at all.

14. A G2P1 (SVDX1) at 12+4 weeks gestation with a BMI of 29 is known to have β-thalassaemia major. She had a splenectomy at the age of 11. Two weeks ago she had 2 units RBC transfused. Her blood results report Hb 106g/l and PLT 623 X 109/L.

15. A G3P2 (SVDX2) at 12+6 weeks gestation with a BMI of 28 is known to have β-thalassaemia major. She had a splenectomy at the age of 12. She had 2 units RBC transfused 2 weeks ago. Her Hb is 106g/l and PLTS 423 X 109/L. She was admitted to hospital with abdominal pain.

16. A G3P2 (SVDX2) at 35+4 weeks gestation with a BMI of 27 is known to have β-thalassaemia major. She had undergone a splenectomy at the age of 10. Her Hb is 76g/l, she is asymptomatic of anaemia and has got normal foetal growth.

Options for questions 17 - 20

A. Immediately
B. 3 days
C. 5 days
D. 7 days
E. 10 days
F. 2 weeks
G. 3 weeks
H. 4 weeks
I. 6 weeks
J. 3 months
K. 4 months
L. 6 months
M. 12 months
N. No need
O. At the time of mifepristone administration
P. At the time of misoprostol administration
Q. After uterine cavity has been emptied

Instructions

For each clinical scenario below, choose the single most appropriate option from the list. Each option maybe used once, more than once, or not at all.

17. A 21-year-old lady had a normal vaginal delivery yesterday. She would like to know when to commence contraception. She is not going to breastfeed.

18. A 34-year-old lady had a normal delivery a few hours ago. She would like to know when is the soonest she could have a Mirena coil fitted in?

19. A 31-year-old lady had an emergency C-section this morning for failure to progress at 8 cm. She is asking when is the earliest she could have a progesterone-only implant fitted, as she would like one as soon as possible?

20. A 41-year-old lady had a vaginal delivery a few weeks ago. She had a condom failure last night and is requesting emergency contraception. She is unable to swallow oral medication. How soon after delivery is a Cu-IUD safe to be used as emergency contraception?

Options for questions 21 - 22

A. No need for anti-D

B. Give 250 IU anti-D

C. Give 250 IU anti-D and request Kleihauer

D. Discuss with hematology lab how much extra anti-D is needed

E. Give 500 IU anti-D

F. Give 500 IU anti-D and request Kleihauer

G. Give 500 IU anti-D and request Kleihauer, both within 72 hours from delivery

H. Give 500 IU anti-D and request Kleihauer, both within 72 hours from diagnosis of IUD

I. Give 1500 IU anti-D

J. Request cffDNA

K. None of the above

Instructions

For each clinical scenario below, choose the single most appropriate management option from the list. Each option maybe used once, more than once, or not at all.

21. A 31-year-old G2P1 Rhesus negative, non-sensitised lady who was at 24 weeks gestation presented with vaginal bleeding. She had a placenta praevia confirmed at her anomaly scan and received 500 IU Anti-D Ig. Kleihauer indicated a further FMH of approximately 2ml.

22. A 41-year-old G1P0 presented at 31 weeks gestation. She was a non-sensitised Rhesus negative lady who received RAADP at 29 weeks with a dose of 1500 IU anti-D Ig. She was in a high impact RTA and is wondering what should be done.

Options for questions 23 - 26

    A. PDS 3-0 on a curved 31mm needle

    B. PDS 2-0 on a curved 36mm needle

    C. PDS 1 on a curved 36mm needle

    D. Vicryl rapide 3-0 on a curved 26mm needle

    E. Vicryl rapide 2-0 on a curved 36mm needle

    F. Vicryl size 1 on a curved 70mm needle

    G. Vicryl size 1 on a curved 40mm needle

    H. Vicryl 2-0 on a curved 31mm needle

    I. Vicryl 3-0 on a curved 26mm needle

    J. Chromic catgut 2-0 on a curved 26mm needle

    K. Mersilk 2-0 on a straight 55mm needle

    L. Prolene 2-0 with a straight 60mm needle

    M. Monocryl 3-0 with a straight 60mm needle

    N. Steri-strip 3mm x 75mm.

    O. Mersilene tape, double-armed 65mm needles

Instructions

For each case below, choose the single most appropriate suture type from the list. Each option maybe used once, more than once, or not at all:

23. To close the rectal mucosa in a 4th degree tear.

24. Cervical cerclage.

25. Brace (B-Lynch) suture.

26. To approximate the external anal sphincter muscle in a 3rd degree tear.

Options for questions 27 - 29

A. Deliver with forceps
B. Perform Lovset's manoeuvre
C. Perform Mauriceau-Smellie-Veit manoeuvre
D. Augment
E. Offer IOL
F. Offer ECV
G. Discuss options
H. Perform USS and offer IOL
I. Perform USS and discuss options
J. Discuss options and perform C/S
K. Start syntocinon infusion
L. Perform FBS
M. Consider C/S
N. Perform C/S
O. Assisted vaginal breech delivery
P. Perform Zavanelli manouvre

Obstetrics paper 1 – Questions

Instructions

For each clinical scenario below, choose the single most appropriate management option from the list. Each option maybe used once, more than once, or not at all.

27. A 25-year-old G2P1 with a previous vaginal delivery is now 37+2 weeks gestation. Her BMI is 34 and she is in spontaneous labour. She ruptured her membranes three hours ago, she is contracting 3:10 minutes and the cervix is 4cm dilated. Her midwife has called you to assess presentation as she thought the presenting part was breech. You confirmed this by ultrasound.

28. A 28-year-old G2P1 with a previous vaginal delivery four years ago is now 38+2 weeks pregnant. Her BMI is 28 and she presented in spontaneous labour. She has got a date for elective C/S for breech presentation at 39 weeks. Baby is still breech on USS assessment which you performed. Labour is progressing well and cervix is now 6 cm dilated. There are variable decelerations on CTG.

29. A 30-year-old G2P1 with one previous vaginal delivery is now 40+10 weeks gestation. She was under midwifery-led care until you were called to see her and confirmed frank breech presentation at 7 cm dilation. She is keen for vaginal delivery and she has just ruptured her membranes.

Options for questions 30 - 31

A. 250 iu anti-D

B. 500 iu anti-D

C. 1000 iu anti-D

D. 1500 iu anti-D

E. 3000 iu anti-D

F. Kleihauer test in 1 week

G. 250 iu anti-D + Kleihauer test

H. 500 iu anti-D + Kleihauer test

I. 1000 iu anti-D + Kleihauer test

J. 1500 iu anti-D + Kleihauer test

K. 3000 iu anti-D + Kleihauer test

L. Omit anti-D

M. No anti-D required

Instructions

For each clinical scenario below, choose the single most appropriate management option from the list. Each option maybe used once, more than once, or not at all.

30. A 26-year-old lady, G1P0 at 36+3 weeks gestation attended ECV clinic and breech presentation was confirmed by USS. She was AB blood group, Rh negative. ECV was successful. She had no vaginal bleeding after the procedure and CTG was normal.

31. A 40-year-old G5P4 (4 normal vaginal deliveries) at 36 weeks gestation attends after having been involved in a low impact road traffic accident where she was the driver. She is Rhesus negative and had anti-D antibodies on her last blood test.

Options for questions 32 - 35

A. Screen for GBS by taking low vaginal swab
B. Screen for GBS by taking high vaginal swab
C. Screen for GBS at 35 – 37 weeks
D. Screen for GBS at 32 – 34 weeks
E. Offer testing for GBS or intrapartum antibiotics
F. Prescribe benzylpenicillin
G. Prescribe cephalosporins
H. Prescribe benzylpenicillin in labour
I. Prescribe vancomycin
J. Prescribe vancomycin in labour
K. Prescribe antibiotics to treat GBS now and in labour
L. Avoid sweeping the membranes
M. Perform vaginal cleansing in labour
N. Expedite delivery
O. Vaginal delivery is contraindicated

Instructions

For each clinical scenario below, select the single most appropriate management option from the list. Each option maybe used once, more than once, or not at all.

32. A 28-year-old G2P1 with DCDA twins at booking visit is enquiring what measures will be taken in this pregnancy, in light of a history of GBS in her previous pregnancy.

33. A 33-year-old G3P1 at 12 weeks gestation comes to the booking clinic. She had a baby with late-onset GBS disease and is wondering if this will affect care during labour this time.

34. A 30-year-old G1P0 has a sister whose baby was affected with GBS. She would like to be screened.

35. An 18-year-old G1P0 attended the obstetric assessment unit at 22 weeks with abdominal pain. Following urine dipstick assessment, a mid-stream urine sample has been sent off at your request. Three days later the result is reported as GBS positive with 2 X 105 cfu/ml.

Options for questions 36 - 40

A. 2500 iu Dalteparin od from 12 weeks + 6/52 PN

B. 2500 iu Dalteparin bd from 12 weeks

C. 2500 iu Dalteparin bd from 12 weeks + 10/7 PN

D. 2500 iu Dalteparin bd from 28 weeks + 10/7 PN

E. 2500 iu Dalteparin bd from 12 weeks + 6/52 PN

F. 2500 iu Dalteparin bd from 28 weeks + 6/52 PN

G. 5000 iu Dalteparin od

H. 5000 iu Dalteparin bd

I. 5000 iu Dalteparin bd + 10/7 PN

J. 5000 iu Dalteparin od + 6/52 PN

K. 20 mg Enoxaparin bd + 6/52 PN

L. 40 mg Enoxaparin bd

M. 60 mg Enoxaparin od

N. 60 mg Enoxaparin od from 12 weeks + 10/7 PN

O. 60 mg Enoxaparin od from 12 weeks + 6/52 PN

P. 60 mg Enoxaparin od from 28 weeks + 6/52 PN

Q. 60 mg Enoxaparin bd

R. 9000 iu Tinzaparin od

S. 9000 iu Tinzaparin bd

T. Stockings

U. Mobilization and avoidance of dehydration

V. No need for thromboprophylaxis

Obstetrics paper 1 – Questions

Instructions

For each clinical scenario below, choose the single most appropriate option from the list. Each option maybe used once, more than once, or not at all.

36. A 37-year-old G4P3 (SVDX3) is now 12 weeks pregnant and weighs 101 kg. She is a smoker in a wheelchair and is pregnant with twins.

37. A 21-year-old lady who has one child is now 7+ weeks pregnant and weighs 54 kg. This is an IVF pregnancy with OHSS.

38. A 31-year-old lady G3P2 is 11+ weeks pregnant and weighs 62 kg. She was admitted to hospital because her inflammatory bowel disease was "playing up" and she needed her medication changed.

39. A 31-year-old para 1 is 12+ weeks pregnant. She weighs 92 kg with a BMI of 32. She is suffering with inflammatory bowel disease and is complaining of painful varicose veins.

40. A 15-year-old girl is nulliparous and 8 weeks pregnant. Her weight is 56 kg. She has a UTI with a temperature of 37.7° C and was admitted with vomiting.

Options for questions 41 - 43

A. Stillbirth
B. Neonatal death
C. Late foetal loss
D. Extended perinatal death
E. Maternal death
F. Maternity
G. Ectopic pregnancy
H. Early foetal loss
I. Maternal mortality ratio
J. Late maternal death
K. Direct maternal death
L. Indirect maternal death
M. Maternal mortality rate
N. Coincidental death during pregnancy

Instructions

For each clinical scenario below, select the most appropriate classification from the list. Each option maybe used once, more than once, or not at all.

41. A pregnant lady attended the obstetric assessment unit at 25 weeks gestation reporting decreased foetal movements. No foetal heart sounds were detected with a Sonicaid and this was confirmed with an ultrasound scan. She went on to have a normal vaginal delivery.

42. A 25-year old presented at 28 weeks gestation to delivery suite with a placental abruption. The baby was delivered by Caesarean section and handed over to the paediatric team. Unfortunately, 2 days later the baby died.

43. A 23+0 week pregnant lady presented to the obstetric assessment unit with green discharge and painful contractions. She went on to deliver a foetus with no signs of life.

Options for questions 44 - 45

    A. 2-5 in 1000 procedures in 10 years

    B. Up to 15% of bowel injuries might not be diagnosed at the time of surgery

    C. 1 in 10

    D. 1 in 20

    E. 4 in 100

    F. 9 in 100

    G. 11 in 100

    H. 21 in 100

    I. 3-6 in 1000

    J. 1 in 2000

Instructions

When obtaining consent for an obstetric procedure, outline the operative risk that you would quote to the patient in each clinical scenario below. Each option maybe used once, more than once, or not at all.

44. The risk of hysterectomy in a G1P0 who is having elective Caesarean section for placenta praevia.

45. The risk of extensive vaginal tear with vacuum delivery of the foetus.

Options for questions 46 - 50

A. Aspirin

B. Aspirin and cervical cerclage

C. Aspirin and clexane

D. Aspirin and clexane and cervical length measurement

E. betaHCG supplements

F. Cervical cerclage at 14 weeks

G. Cervical cerclage at 16 weeks

H. USS for cervical length

I. USS for cervical length and foetal fibronectin test

J. Vaginal progesterone

K. Offer choice of cervical cerclage or vaginal progesterone

L. Foetal fibronectin test

M. Observe

N. Refer to midwifery-led care

O. Refer to pre-implantation genetic screening

Obstetrics paper 1 – Questions

Instructions

For each clinical scenario below, choose the single most appropriate management option from the list. Each option maybe used once, more than once, or not at all.

46. A 22-year-old G2P0+1 attends your ANC at 12 weeks gestation. You review her medical notes which reveal a miscarriage 3 years ago at 22+3 weeks.

47. A 32-year-old G2P1 (SVD at 35 weeks 2 years ago) presents to the obstetric assessment unit at 27+6 weeks with vaginal pressure symptoms. You perform a speculum examination and see that the cervix is dilated with bulging membranes and a foot that is visible, descending through the cervix.

48. A 22-year-old G3P2 (SVD X 2 at term) at 31 weeks gestation presents to the obstetric assessment unit with irregular, painful, palpable contractions. Speculum examination reveals a closed cervix. She has no history of SROM/PPROM. CTG is normal and urine dipstick showed one plus of ketones.

49. A 29-year-old G2P2 (twins delivered vaginally at 37 weeks) at 32 weeks gestation presents to the obstetric assessment unit with irregular, painful, palpable contractions. Speculum examination reveals a closed cervix. She has no history of SROM/PPROM. CTG is normal and the urine dipstick showed one plus of ketones. You offer her a transvaginal scan to measure the cervical length but she declines.

50. A 27-year-old G2P0+1 had a late miscarriage at 23 weeks, several years ago. Placental microscopy showed multiple infarctions throughout. Blood tests performed at the time revealed abnormally high anti-cardiolipin antibodies. The patient was diagnosed with CIN 3 at her first smear test for which she has undergone a LLETZ procedure. Reviewing the records an 8 mm excision depth was performed. She attends your antenatal clinic at 12+2 weeks gestation for review.

Gynaecology paper 2 - Questions

Options for questions 1 – 5

    A. Colposcopy

    B. Colposcopy + biopsy

    C. Cease recall for age reasons

    D. Colposcopy, see and treat

    E. Cytology at 6 months

    F. Gynaecology referral

    G. HPV test

    H. MDT

    I. Routine recall

    J. Hysterectomy

    K. LLETZ

    L. Cone biopsy

    M. High vaginal swab

    N. No need for cervical smear

Instructions

For each clinical scenario below, choose the single most appropriate management option from the list. Each option maybe used once, more than once, or not at all.

1. A 31-year-old lady who had a normal smear one year ago and no history of smear pathology is in GUM with post-coital bleeding and genital warts.

2. A 25-year-old woman with MRKH syndrome who is sexually active.

3. A 38-year-old lady who had high-grade dyskariosis reported on her last smear.

4. A 25-year-old woman who had some bleeding when the nurse took her smear sample.

5. A 50-year-old lady attended for her first ever smear after learning she had been exposed to diethylstilbestrol (DES) in utero.

Options for questions 6 - 9

  A. Abdominal hysterectomy
  B. COCP
  C. GnRH analogue
  D. Jaydess IUS
  E. POP
  F. Lifestyle advice
  G. LNG IUS
  H. Norethisterone
  I. Tranexamic acid
  J. Mefenamic acid
  K. Endometrial ablation
  L. Supra-cervical laparoscopic hysterectomy
  M. Uterine artery embolisation
  N. Vaginal hysterectomy
  O. Yasmin
  P. None of the above

Instructions

Select the most appropriate treatment for each clinical case outlined below.

6. A 32-year-old para 2 presents to gynaecology clinic with menorrhagia. Her family is complete.

7. A 45-year-old lady presents with menorrhagia, she is a para 8 (8 x SVD), has a BMI of 68 and requires a wheelchair to mobilise due to severe osteoarthritis. OP hysteroscopy was normal and a pipelle biopsy reports endometrial hyperplasia without atypia.

8. A 45-year-old presents to gynaecology clinic with menorrhagia. She is a para 4 (4 x SVDs), has a BMI of 69 and severe COPD, which has required two ITU admissions in the last year. A pipelle biopsy reports endometrial hyperplasia with atypia.

9. A 51-year-old lady presents to gynaecology clinic with menorrhagia and occasional inter-menstrual bleeding. She is nulliparous and has a BMI of 36. Her past operative history includes uterine ventral suspension for primary infertility and a sigmoid colectomy for recurrent dysplastic polyps and subsequent midline incisional hernia repair with synthetic mesh. You obtained an endometrial biopsy and the histology reports endometrial hyperplasia with atypia.

Options for questions 10 - 11

A. Appendicitis
B. Bladder pain syndrome
C. Diverticulitis
D. Ectopic pregnancy
E. Endometriosis
F. Ovarian cyst torsion
G. Over active bladder
H. Pelvic congestion syndrome
I. Pelvic inflammatory disease
J. Renal stone
K. Ruptured ovarian cyst
L. Urodynamic stress incontinence
M. Urinary tract infection
N. None of the above

Instructions

For each clinical scenario below, choose the single most likely diagnosis from the list. Each option maybe used once, more than once, or not at all.

10. A 17-year-old girl presents to the emergency gynaecology clinic with generalized pelvic pain (no lateralizing symptoms). She also has urinary frequency, dysuria and a blood stained, brown vaginal discharge. She has a new boyfriend and they are using condoms for contraception. Her last period was two weeks ago. Her urine hCG is negative.

11. A 58-year-old lady presents to A&E with left-sided pelvic pain which has been present for two weeks but has worsened in the last two days. She went through the menopause at the age of 50. She is not sexually active. She has a past medical history of irritable bowel syndrome. Her past operative history includes laparoscopic left salpingo-oophorectomy for a dermoid cyst (10 years ago.) Urinalysis is negative.

Options for questions 12 - 14

    A. Lifestyle advice
    B. Vaginal oestrogen pessary
    C. Vaginal oestrogen ring
    D. Oestrogen implant
    E. Continuous combined HRT
    F. Sequential HRT
    G. Topical oestrogen
    H. Oestrogen and progesterone patch
    I. Topical oestrogen and Mirena IUS
    J. Testosterone gel
    K. Testosterone implant
    L. Fluoxetine
    M. Black cohosh
    N. St John's Wort
    O. Cognitive behavioural therapy

Instructions

For each clinical scenario below, choose the single most appropriate management option from the list. Each option maybe used once, more than once, or not at all.

12. A 49-year-old lady has been amenorrhoeic for 18 months. She has hot flushes, night sweats and mood swings. She has a BMI of 43. She is struggling to cope and demands HRT. What treatment would you recommend?

13. A 51-year-old lady went through the menopause 5 years ago. She has hot flushes and night sweats. She had breast cancer and right mastectomy 2 years ago, she is taking tamoxifen. What treatment would you recommend?

14. A 35-year-old lady has been diagnosed with premature ovarian insufficiency. What treatment would you recommend?

Options for questions 15 - 19

A. Avoid intercourse
B. Copper coil
C. Too late for emergency contraception
D. Defer oral contraceptive for 5 days
E. Defer oral contraceptive for 7 days
F. Oestrogen
G. LNG oral emergency contraceptive
H. LNG oral emergency contraceptive double dose 3 mg
I. Mirena coil
J. Perform pregnancy test
K. Start oral contraceptive pill
L. UPA oral emergency contraceptive
M. UPA oral emergency contraceptive double dose

Instructions

For each clinical scenario below, select the single most appropriate management option from the list. Each option maybe used once, more than once, or not at all.

15. A 34-year-old lady had unprotected intercourse 48 hours ago. She is taking St John's Wort for depression and is on the waiting list for a trachelectomy for cervical cancer. What emergency contraception would be most suitable for her?

16. A 24 year-old-lady attended family planning clinic for emergency contraception. She had UPSI yesterday, on day 20, of her cycle. Her periods are usually 31 day cycles.

17. An 18-year-old girl who has a BMI of 34 had UPSI 3 days ago, which was day 8 of her cycle. She would like emergency contraception but tells you that she previously passed out when her GP attempted to insert a Mirena coil. She took LNG-EC 6 days ago from the pharmacy.

18. A 21-year-old lady had UPSI 2 days ago on day 10 of her 30 day cycle. She is not keen on having an IUCD inserted due to a past history of chlamydia. She has been taking the mini pill sporadically.

19. A 32-year-old lady attended A&E for EC because she was sexually assaulted 5 days ago. Her period is due in 2 days time.

Options for questions 20 - 22

A. Clomiphene citrate
B. Eflornithine (topical)
C. Gonadotrophin therapy
D. Laparoscopic ovarian diathermy
E. Letrozole
F. Lifestyle changes
G. Metformin
H. Mirena IUS
I. Norethisterone (cyclical)
J. NovoRapid
K. Simvastatin
L. Spironolactone
M. Yasmin
N. None of the above

Instructions

For each clinical scenario below, choose the single most appropriate treatment option from the list. Each option maybe used once, more than once, or not at all.

20. A 24-year-lady with PCOS has anovulatory infertility. She has a BMI of 22, an elevated serum LH and free androgen index. She completed 6 cycles of clomiphene citrate but failed to ovulate.

21. A 25-year-old lady with PCOS has irregular periods and primary infertility. She has a BMI of 24 and an elevated LH. She completed 6 cycles of clomiphene citrate but has just moved to a house 80 miles away from the nearest hospital.

22. A 28-year-old lady with PCOS and anovulatory infertility is receiving gonadotrophin therapy. After hCG administration to trigger ovulation she develops one follicle with a 19mm diameter and four follicles which are greater than 14mm in diameter.

Options for questions 23 - 25

A. Check karyotype

B. Perform test for Fragile X permutation

C. Check for 21-OH antibodies and TPO antibodies

D. Perform diabetes screening

E. Perform infection screening

F. Refer to cardiologist, geneticist and endocrinologist

G. Book for gonadectomy

H. Commence POP

I. Arrange DEXA scan annually

J. Arrange DEXA scan 5 yearly

Instructions

For each clinical scenario below, choose the single most appropriate management option from the list. Each option maybe used once, more than once, or not at all.

23. A 20-year-old lady presents to gynaecology clinic with sporadic periods since the age of 16. The last one was 6 months ago. Her BMI is 30 and FSH taken at her last consultation is 31. Karyotype is XO.

24. You reviewed a 35-year-old lady in your gynaecology clinic following investigation for suspected POI. You have commenced her on hormone replacement therapy.

25. A 33-year-old lady presents with absent periods for 17 months. The FSH level done by her GP is 49. She is fit and well and has never had any surgery. She has a 6 year old son with learning difficulties.

Options for questions 26 - 28

A. 2-5:1000 procedures in 10 years

B. Up to 15% of bowel injuries might not be diagnosed at the time of surgery

C. 1 in 10

D. 1 in 20

E. 4 in 100

F. 9 in 100

G. 11 in 100

H. 21 in 100

I. 3-6 in 1000

J. 1 in 2000

K. None of the above

Instructions

For each procedure below, choose the single most appropriate option from the list. Each option maybe used once, more than once, or not at all.

26. Failure rate for sterilisation by vasectomy.

27. Risk of persistent trophoblastic tissue with laparoscopic salpingotomy.

28. Need for repeat surgical procedure following surgical evacuation of uterus.

Options for questions 29 - 32

A. Kelly plication
B. Marshall-Marchetti-Krantz procedure
C. Paravaginal deficit repair
D. Urodynamics
E. Refer to tertiary centre
F. MDT
G. Botox A
H. Percutaneous sacral nerve stimulation
I. Autologous rectus fascial sling
J. Duloxetine
K. Desmopressin
L. Oxybutynin
M. Mirabegron
N. Tolterodine
O. Darifenacin
P. Oestrogen cream vaginally
Q. Percutaneous posterior tibial nerve stimulation
R. Pad test

Gynaecology Paper 2 – Questions

Instructions

For each clinical scenario below, choose the single most likely management option from the list. Each option maybe used once, more than once, or not at all.

29. A 46-year-old lady has been referred to clinic with worsening nocturia, needing to void 3-4 times during the night. Her GP prescribed tolterodine 6 months ago but this had little benefit. She avoids drinking after 7pm. She is fit and well and has not had previous surgery. She has 3 children, all delivered vaginally.

30. A 52-year-old lady returns to your gynaecology clinic with recurrent stress urinary incontinence. She had a Marshall-Marchetti-Krantz procedure 18 years ago. She would like to run a marathon next year but finds it impossible to train as she leaks when running.

31. A 68-year-old lady is referred by her GP because she has to rush to the toilet all the time. If she does not set an alarm clock to wake her 3 times in the night she will wet her bed in the morning. She has tried a number of pharmacological treatments but nothing has helped. On examination you find that her BMI is 26 and she has moderate anterior vaginal wall prolapse.

32. A 65-year-old lady is suffering with overactive bladder symptoms. She has tried numerous oral treatments, including mirabegron, with minimal effect. She has severe arthritis and finds it difficult to mobilize. When you discuss botox injections and explain the risk of self-catheterisation she is not keen to proceed due to her physical constraints.

Options for questions 33 - 34

A. 1
B. 2
C. 3
D. 4
E. 5
F. 6
G. 8
H. 9
I. 10
J. 12
K. 15
L. 20
M. 24
N. 25

Instructions

For each clinical scenario below, choose the single most appropriate option from the list. Each option maybe used once, more than once, or not at all.

33. An 89-year-old lady with a BMI of 60 presented to gynaecology clinic with post-menopausal bleeding. She has had three non-STEMI's in the past twelve months. You skillfully obtained an endometrial biopsy and the histology reports endometrial hyperplasia without atypia. She is keen to commence oral progestogens and asks when a repeat endometrial biopsy will be performed (in months)?

34. An 87-year-old lady with a BMI of 58 presented to gynaecology clinic with post-menopausal bleeding. She has had three myocardial infarctions and a CABG was performed one month ago. You successfully obtained an endometrial biopsy and the histology reports endometrial hyperplasia with atypia. She declines a hysterectomy but agrees to commence oral progestogens. When should you offer to repeat endometrial surveillance (in months)?

Gynaecology Paper 2 – Questions

Options for questions 35 - 37

A. Ultrasound scan

B. Discharge from follow up

C. Laparoscopy

D. Laparoscopy and oophorectomy

E. Laparoscopy and de-torsion of the ovary

F. Laparotomy

G. Oophoropexy

H. Consider MRI

I. Consider CT

J. CA 125

K. CA 125, LDH

L. CA 125, LDH, bHCG, AFP

Instructions

For each clinical scenario below, choose the single most important management option from the list. Each option maybe used once, more than once, or not at all.

35. A 15-year-old girl who presented to A&E with left iliac fossa pain was diagnosed with mittelschmertz, as her last period was 2 weeks ago. A pelvic ultrasound scan reports a simple ovarian cyst measuring 8 cm on the right ovary.

36. A 15-year-old girl has been menstruating regularly for 4 years and is referred to your clinic for review. She was being investigated by her GP for chronic constipation. On pelvic ultrasound scan it was reported that she had a 4 cm complex cyst on the left ovary. There was no free fluid in the Pouch of Douglas.

37. A 14-year-old girl has attended clinic following a pelvic ultrasound scan which has shown a persistent simple cyst that has grown 2 cm in size since the last scan. It is now measuring 7 cm. She has no symptoms.

Options for questions 38 - 40

A. Bowen's disease of vulva
B. Herpes simplex infection
C. HSIL of vulva
D. Human papillomavirus infection
E. Lichen planus
F. Lichen sclerosus
G. Lichen simplex
H. LSIL of vulva
I. Vulval candidiasis
J. Vulval eczema
K. Vulval intraepithelial neoplasia
L. Vulval psoriasis
M. Provoked vulvodynia
N Unprovoked vulvodynia

Instructions

For each clinical scenario below, choose the single most likely diagnosis/appropriate treatment option from the list. Each option maybe used once, more than once, or not at all.

38. A 29-year-old lady presents to gynaecology clinic with a two year history of vulval pain which she describes as a severe, burning sensation at the introitus which occurs at penetration when having sexual intercourse. She reports recurrent episodes of vulvo-vaginal candidiasis which respond well to oral fluconazole. On examination the vulva and vagina appear entirely normal, there is normal sensation with localized tenderness (to light touch) at the introitus.

39. An 89-year-old lady presents to gynaecology clinic with recurrent urinary tract infections and poor urinary flow for the past two years. She also describes generalized vulval soreness. She has not been sexually active since her husband died 24 years ago. She has no relevant past medical history. On examination of the vulva the skin appears pale, white and atrophic, there is complete labial fusion with only a pinhole opening draining urine.

40. A 62-year-old lady attends gynaecology clinic with a longstanding history of vulval itch and soreness. She describes superficial and deep dyspareunia often with post-coital bleeding and a recurrent blood stained discharge. On further questioning she denies any past dermatological conditions but reports painful gums and recurrent mouth ulcers. On examination, inspection of the mouth finds white patches on the insides of the cheeks and several ulcers. A vulval exam finds the labia minora have bright red, eroded surfaces with Wickham's striae at the epithelial border. Gentle digital examination finds multiple vaginal synechiae.

Options for questions 41 - 44

A. Amitriptyline
B. Cimetidine
C. Desmopressin
D. Duloxetine

E. Gabapentin
F. Intravesical bacillus Calmette-Guerin
G. Intravesical lidocaine

H. Intravesical resiniferatoxin
I. Mirabegron
J. Oxybutynin IR
K. Posterior tibial nerve stimulation
L. Sacral neuromodulation
M. Tolterodine

N. None of the above

Instructions

For each clinical scenario below, choose the most appropriate treatment option from the list. Each option maybe used once, more than once, or not at all.

41. A 59-year-old lady presented to the urogynaecology clinic with overactive bladder symptoms. She has tried bladder training and oxybutynin, darifenacin then mirabegron, with limited efficacy. Urodynamics reported detrusor overactivity. She couldn't tolerate cystoscopy for regular botulinum toxin injections and was keen for a more definitive treatment. What treatment option would you discuss next?

42. An 89-year-old lady presents to the urogynaecology clinic with a longstanding history of urinary urgency with incontinence, frequency of up to 20 episodes per day and nocturia. She has a BMI of 17 and is very frail. Her pelvic examination reveals no evidence of prolapse or demonstrable stress incontinence.

43. A 54-year-old lady presents to the urogynaecology clinic with urinary frequency and urge incontinence with nocturia of 4 episodes per night. She attended the continence advisor and lifestyle changes have greatly improved her daytime symptoms. Unfortunately there has been little improvement in the nocturia. She has no current medical problems and is not taking any medication.

44. A 48-year-old lady presents to the urogynaecology clinic with symptoms of worsening stress incontinence. She is a para 1, vaginal delivery, and she has a BMI of 21. She has attended 6 months of physiotherapy and pelvic floor exercises have improved but not resolved her symptoms. She refuses any surgical intervention and wants to know what treatment options you can offer her?

Options for questions 45 - 46

A. Complete androgen insensitivity syndrome

B. Congenital adrenal hyperplasia

C. Fragile X syndrome

D. Imperforate hymen

E. Klinefelter syndrome

F. Kallmann syndrome

G. McCune-Albright syndrome

H. Mayer-Rokitansky-Küster-Hauser (MRKH)

I. Partial androgen insensitivity syndrome

J. Swyer syndrome

K. Transverse lower vaginal septum

L. Turner syndrome

Instructions
For each clinical scenario below, choose the single most likely diagnosis. Each option maybe used once, more than once, or not at all.

45. A 15-year-old girl presents with primary amenorrhoea and no secondary sexual characteristics. Blood investigations show low GnRH, FSH and LH levels. She has difficulty distinguishing the smell of coffee, cinnamon and cloves.

46. A 16-year-old girl presents with short stature and delayed onset of puberty. Ultrasound scans revealed small uterus and small ovaries. On examination she has a webbed neck, low set ears with a broad chest and widely spaced nipples.

Options for questions 47 - 50

A. Cyclical use of drospirenone-containing COC

B. Continuous use of drospirenone-containing COC

C. Percutaneous estradiol and progestogen

D. Micronised progesterone

E. Danazol 200 mg BD

F. GnRH analogues

G. GnRH analogue and tibolone

H. Progesterone

I. LNG-IUS

J. Spironolactone

K. Hysterectomy and bilateral salpingo-oophorectomy

L. Hysterectomy with conservation of ovaries

M. Vitex agnus castus

N. Fluoxetine in luteal phase

O. SSRI in luteal phase

P. Endometrial ablation

Instructions

For each clinical scenario below, choose the single most appropriate management option from the list. Each option maybe used once, more than once, or not at all.

47. A 32-year-old lady has been referred by her GP with menorrhagia. On further questioning her predominant symptoms are of a cyclical low mood with extreme volatility and irritability that improve with menstruation. Her menorrhagia has improved with tranexamic acid. What treatment option would you recommend?

48. A 39-year-old lady has returned to PMS clinic for review after your prescription of GnRH analogues and tibolone, which you gave her 6 months ago. She is also known to have adenomyosis. She feels like a new woman, reports good mood, her pelvic pain is gone and she has even started having intercourse with her husband again. What is the next step?

49. A 34-year-old lady has been referred by her GP with lack of concentration, low mood, irritability, breast tenderness, bloating and feeling as if she has lost control. She has tried CBT and continuous COC without any improvement. You review her Daily Record of Severity of Problems over the last 3 months. There is no obvious cyclical pattern. What is the next step?

50. A 29-year-old lady attended with her male partner. He complains that she is really moody and 10 days before her period is due she becomes aggressive, to the extent where she throws plates at him. The lady reveals that her GP has not tried any medication but referred her for CBT only, which did not help.

Obstetrics paper 2 - Questions

Options for questions 1 – 4

A. Aspirin

B. Aspirin and cervical cerclage

C. Aspirin and Clexane

D. Aspirin and Clexane and cervical length measurement

E. betaHCG supplements

F. Cervical cerclage at 14 weeks

G. Cervical cerclage at 16 weeks

H. USS for cervical length

I. USS for cervical length and foetal fibronectin test

J. Vaginal progesterone

K. Offer choice of cervical cerclage or vaginal progesterone

L. Foetal fibronectin test

M. Observe

N. Refer to midwifery-led care

O. Refer to pre-implantation genetic screening

Instructions

For each clinical scenario below, choose the single most appropriate management option from the list. Each option maybe used once, more than once, or not at all.

1. A 31-year-old G2P0+1 presents to your antenatal clinic for her booking appointment. She had a miscarriage at 21 weeks gestation, 4 years ago. On questioning she reveals that she underwent a LLETZ procedure for CIN3 after her first smear. Histology from her colposcopy record shows an excision depth of 17 mm was performed.

2. A 32-year-old G2P0+1 attends your antenatal clinic at 28 weeks gestation. She has a history of miscarriage at 21 weeks. You were monitoring her cervical length which was 32 mm at 24 weeks. An SHO has requested cervical length measurement at 28 weeks which was 21 mm.

3. A 29-year-old lady in her first pregnancy was referred to your ANC by her midwife because she had cone biopsy preformed following a diagnosis of CIN3. Report following the excision showed that 19 mm deep cone biopsy was excised. Her smear is now normal and she is 16 weeks pregnant with a cervical length of 22 mm on the scan today.

4. A 19-year-old G2P1 attends your ANC at 20 weeks of gestation following her anomaly scan. She had a normal vaginal delivery at 35 weeks previously following PPROM at 29 weeks gestation.

Options for questions 5 – 8

A. 2500 iu Dalteparin od from 12 weeks + 6/52 PN
B. 2500 iu Dalteparin bd from 12 weeks
C. 2500 iu Dalteparin bd from 12 weeks + 10/7 PN
D. 2500 iu Dalteparin bd from 28 weeks + 10/7 PN
E. 2500 iu Dalteparin bd from 12 weeks + 6/52 PN
F. 2500 iu Dalteparin bd from 28 weeks + 6/52 PN
G. 5000 iu Dalteparin od
H. 5000 iu Dalteparin bd
I. 5000 iu Dalteparin bd + 10/7 PN
J. 5000 iu Dalteparin od + 6/52 PN
K. 20 mg Enoxaparin bd + 6/52 PN
L. 40 mg Enoxaparin bd
M. 60 mg Enoxaparin od
N. 60 mg Enoxaparin od from 12 weeks + 10/7 PN
O. 60 mg Enoxaparin od from 12 weeks + 6/52 PN
P. 60 mg Enoxaparin od from 28 weeks + 6/52 PN
Q. 60 mg Enoxaparin bd
R. 9000 iu Tinzaparin od
S. 9000 iu Tinzaparin bd
T. Stockings
U. Mobilization and avoidance of dehydration
V. No need for thromboprophylaxis

Instructions

For each clinical scenario below, choose the single most appropriate option from the list. Each option maybe used once, more than once, or not at all.

5. An 18-year-old girl is nulliparous and has just discovered that she is 8 weeks pregnant. She weighs 120 kg and her BMI is 45. She had a PE after an appendicectomy 6 years ago.

6. A 22-year-old woman has one child and is 5+ weeks pregnant. Her weight is 69 kg. She is taking warfarin for antithrombin deficiency as she suffered two previous DVTs and a PE four years ago.

7. A 24-year-old woman who is P0 is 12+ weeks pregnant. She weighs 49 kg. She uses illegal substances intravenously and has got heterozygous factor V Leiden disease.

8. A 34-year-old G4P2 is 26 weeks pregnant. Her weight is 95 kg with a BMI of 38. She has extensive lower limb varicose veins and has developed early PET.

Options for questions 9 - 10

A. Deliver with forceps

B. Perform Lovset's manoeuvre

C. Perform Mauriceau-Smellie-Veit manoeuvre

D. Augment

E. Offer IOL

F. Offer ECV

G. Discuss options

H. Perform USS and offer IOL

I. Perform USS and discuss options

J. Discuss options and perform C/S

K. Start syntocinon infusion

L. Perform FBS

M. Consider C/S

N. Perform C/S

O. Assisted vaginal breech delivery

P. Perform Zavanelli manouvre

Instructions

For each clinical scenario below, choose the single most appropriate management option from the list. Each option maybe used once, more than once, or not at all.

9. An 18-year-old G1P0 presented at 38+3 weeks gestation in labour with a frank breech presentation. She is making good progress with labour but the after-coming head has still not delivered 3 minutes following delivery of the shoulders.

10. A 38-year-old G3P2 at 38 weeks gestation is wheeled into a labour room by an ambulance crew. She was planning to have home delivery but the midwife assessed her at home and found a breech presentation. You confirm a frank breech presentation on USS and a vaginal assessment reveals that she is 9 cm dilated.

Options for questions 11 - 12

A. No need for anti-D

B. Give 250 IU anti-D

C. Give 250 IU anti-D and request Kleihauer

D. Discuss with the haematology lab how much extra anti-D is needed

E. Give 500 IU anti-D

F. Give 500 IU anti-D and request Kleihauer

G. Give 500 IU anti-D and request Kleihauer, both within 72 hours from delivery

H. Give 500 IU anti-D and request Kleihauer, both within 72 hours from diagnosis of IUD

I. Give 1500 IU anti-D

J. Request cffDNA

K. None of the above

Instructions

For each clinical scenario below, choose the single most appropriate management option from the list. Each option maybe used once, more than once, or not at all.

11. A 30-year-old G2P1, Rhesus negative lady has anti-D antibodies detected when she presents at 24 weeks gestation. She has a known placenta praevia and continues to bleed intermittently.

12. A 22-year-old G2P0, Rhesus negative, non-sensitised lady was 28 weeks pregnant. She had an IUD confirmed 2 days ago and just had an SVD.

Options for questions 13 - 14

A. Manage in community with regular analgesia

B. Give analgesia within 30 minutes of arrival and give effective analgesia in 1 hour

C. Exchange transfusion

D. Top up transfusion

E. Discuss delivery after 38 weeks

F. Admit

G. Consider admission to critical care unit and therapeutic thromboprophylaxis

H. Prophylactic thromboprophylaxis

I. Thrombolysis

J. MRI

K. Broad spectrum antibiotics

L. Give steroids

M. Observe

Instructions

For each clinical scenario below, choose the most appropriate management option from the list. Each option maybe used once, more than once, or not at all.

13. A 25-year-old woman who is G2P1 at 24+2 weeks gestation is known to have SCD. She has been on aspirin since 12 weeks and presents with tachypnoea, chest pain, cough and SOB. Her CXR is clear, temperature is 37.5°C and respiratory rate 24/min. Her oxygen saturations are 93%.

14. A 28-year-old woman who is G2P1 at 24+2 weeks gestation is known to have SCD. She has been taking aspirin since 12 weeks. She presented to the obstetric assessment unit with tachypnoea, chest pain and SOB. Her respiratory rate is 20/min with oxygen saturations of 97% and her temperature is 37.1°C. A CXR shows a new radio-opaque lesion in the right upper lobe. Her haemoglobin level 3 weeks ago was 9.2 g/l and today is 7.2 g/l.

Options for questions 15 - 17

A. No admission, no treatment, BP once a week, urinary protein analysis once a week.

B. No admission, no treatment, BP once a week, urinary protein analysis once a week, PET bloods.

C. No admission, no treatment, BP 2X per week, urinary protein analysis 2X per week.

D. No admission, treat until BP <140/90, BP 2X per week, urinary protein analysis 2X per week.

E. No admission, treat until BP <150/100, BP 2X per week, urinary protein analysis 2X per week.

F. No admission, treat until BP <150/100, BP 2X per week, urinary protein analysis 2X per week, PET bloods.

G. Admit, treat until BP < 140/90, BP once a day, urinary protein analysis once a week.

H. Admit, treat until BP < 150/100, BP once a day, urinary protein analysis once a week.

I. Admit, treat until BP < 150/100, BP once a day, urinary protein analysis once a week, PET bloods.

J. Admit, treat until BP <140/90, BP 4X daily, urinary protein analysis daily, PET bloods.

K. Admit, treat until BP <150/100, BP 4X daily, urinary protein analysis daily, PET bloods.

Instructions

For each clinical scenario, select the most appropriate management option from the list above. Each option maybe used once, more than once, or not at all.

15. A 29-year-old G1P0 with BMI of 32 and blood pressure measuring 152/106 at 26 weeks gestation has no proteinuria and takes no anti-hypertensive medication.

16. A 27-year-old G1P0 with BMI of 32 and blood pressure measuring 152/106 at 26 weeks gestation has one plus (+) of proteinuria and takes no anti-hypertensive medication.

17. A 32-year-old G1P0 with BMI of 32 and blood pressure measuring 168/115 at 26 weeks gestation has no proteinuria and takes no anti-hypertensive medication.

Options for questions 18 - 20

A. Monitor 4 weekly up to 24 weeks then 2 weekly until delivery

B. Monitor 4 weekly up to 28 weeks then 2 weekly until delivery

C. Refer to foetal medicine for IUT

D. Refer to foetal medicine

E. Monitor by MCA PSV every 2 weeks

F. Monitor by MCA PSV every week

G. Deliver

H. Request cffDNA for foetal genotype at 12 weeks

I. Request cffDNA for foetal genotype at 16 weeks

J. Request cffDNA for foetal genotype at 20 weeks

K. Observe

L. Amniocentesis in 5 weeks time

M. Amniocentesis in 12 weeks time

Instructions

For each clinical scenario below, choose the single most appropriate management option from the list. Each option maybe used once, more than once, or not at all.

18. A G2P1 who is at 33 weeks gestation has got an Anti-c titre of 15.0 and her MCA PSV is 1.8 MoM.

19. A G1P0 has been tested for antibodies and is found to be Rh D negative but has got antibodies present. The father of the child is Rh D+ heterozygote.

20. A G1P0 has been tested for antibodies and is found to be Rh K negative with antibodies present. The father of the baby is Rh K+ heterozygote.

Options for questions 21 - 25

A. Screen for GBS by taking low vaginal swab

B. Screen for GBS by taking high vaginal swab

C. Screen for GBS at 35 – 37 weeks

D. Screen for GBS at 32 – 34 weeks

E. Offer testing for GBS or intrapartum antibiotics

F. Prescribe benzylpenicillin

G. Prescribe cephalosporins

H. Prescribe benzylpenicillin in labour

I. Prescribe vancomycin

J. Prescribe vancomycin in labour

K. Prescribe antibiotics to treat GBS now and in labour

L. Avoid sweeping the membranes

M. Perform vaginal cleansing in labour

N. Expedite delivery

O. Vaginal delivery is contraindicated

Instructions

For each clinical scenario below, select the single most appropriate management option from the list. Each option maybe used once, more than once, or not at all.

21. A 21-year-old G2P1 attended obstetric assessment unit at 27 weeks gestation with vaginal discharge. You took a vaginal swab that came back showing GBS colonisation.

22. A 32-year-old G1P0 presented in threatened preterm labour at 33 weeks gestation. Vaginal assessment reveals that she is 5 cm dilated. The GBS screen she requested at 20 weeks is negative.

23. A 19-year old G2P1 attended obstetric assessment unit at 27 weeks gestation with vaginal discharge. You took a vaginal swab that came back showing GBS colonisation. She is now 41 weeks into her pregnancy and presents in labour. She would like to labour in the birthing pool.

24. A 23-year-old G2P1 with DCDA twins (breech/cephalic) at 34+6 weeks gestation had an incidental finding of GBS growth on a swab at 28 weeks. Today she presented with preterm rupture of membranes.

25. A 42-year-old G3P1 at 12 weeks gestation comes to the booking clinic. She had a baby with late onset GBS disease after her last delivery and is now wondering if this will affect her care during labour this time. She has got a severe allergy to penicillin.

Options for questions 26 - 29

A. PDS 3-0 on a curved 31mm needle

B. PDS 2-0 on a curved 36mm needle

C. PDS 1 on a curved 36mm needle

D. Vicryl rapide 3-0 on a curved 26mm needle

E. Vicryl rapide 2-0 on a curved 36mm needle

F. Vicryl size 1 on a curved 70mm needle

G. Vicryl size 1 on a curved 40mm needle

H. Vicryl 2-0 on a curved 31mm needle

I. Vicryl 3-0 on a curved 26mm needle

J. Chromic catgut 2-0 on a curved 26mm needle

K. Mersilk 2-0 on a straight 55mm needle

L. Prolene 2-0 with a straight 60mm needle

M. Monocryl 3-0 with a straight 60mm needle

N. Steri-strip 3mm x 75mm

O. Mersilene tape, double-armed 65mm needles

Instructions

For each case below, choose the single most appropriate suture type from the list. Each option maybe used once, more than once, or not at all:

26. To close the vaginal mucosa following a right mediolateral episiotomy.

27. Laparoscopic oophoropexy.

28. Is no longer used in clinical practice in the UK.

29. Takes 90 - 120 days to absorb.

Options for questions 30 - 32

A. 250 iu anti-D	H. 500 iu anti-D + Kleihauer test
B. 500 iu anti-D	I. 1000 iu anti-D + Kleihauer test
C. 1000 iu anti-D	J. 1500 iu anti-D + Kleihauer test
D. 1500 iu anti-D	K. 3000 iu anti-D + Kleihauer test
E. 3000 iu anti-D	L. Omit anti-D
F. Kleihauer test in 1 week	M. No anti-D required
G. 250 iu anti-D + Kleihauer test	

Instructions

For each clinical scenario below, choose the single most appropriate management option from the list. Each option maybe used once, more than once, or not at all.

30. A 40-year-old G5P4 (4 normal vaginal deliveries) at 36 weeks gestation attends in labour and has a straight forward vaginal delivery. She is Rhesus negative and had anti-D antibodies on her last blood test. Her new partner is Rh positive with DD genotype. During her last pregnancy she required delivery at 34 weeks gestation for foetal hydrops, with haemolytic disease of the neonate (HDN) confirmed. She is on the waiting list for sterilisation in 6 weeks time. She is refusing anti-D because she is fed up with needles.

31. A 35-year-old lady at 38 weeks gestation just underwent an elective Caesarean section for placenta praevia. There was a 2.5 litre measured blood loss and cell salvage was used. She is known to have Rh negative blood with no antibodies. It was not possible to obtain foetal blood sample from the cord to check for neonatal blood group.

32. A 29-year-old primiparous lady with HELLP syndrome required 3 units of platelets following an emergency Caesarean section. She is known to be Rh negative with no antibodies. The blood bank did not have Rh negative platelets available and hence provided Rh positive platelets.

Options for questions 33 - 35

A. 0.5:100
B. 1:100
C. 2:100
D. 0.5:500
E. 1:500
F. 1:750
G. 2:750
H. 0.5:800
I. 1:800
J. 0.5:1000
K. 1:1000
L. 2:1000
M. 1:1500
N. 2:1500

Instructions

For each clinical scenario below, select the single most likely answer from the statistics above. Each option maybe used once, more than once, or not at all.

33. A 38-year-old primiparous lady presents at 40 weeks gestation in active labour. Vaginal examination finds the cervix to be fully dilated and there is an undiagnosed breech presentation 2cm below the spines. Foetal monitoring shows a normal CTG. Ultrasound scan confirms an extended breech with no evidence of neck hyperextension. You are counselling the patient about the risk of vaginal breech delivery. What is the risk of perinatal mortality with a planned vaginal breech delivery?

34. A 27-year-old primiparous lady presents at 40 weeks gestation in active labour. Abdominal examination finds a cephalic presentation, with vaginal examination finding the cervix to be fully dilated and the vertex at 2cm below the spines. What is the risk of perinatal mortality with a planned cephalic birth?

35. A 31-year-old primiparous lady at 38 weeks gestation has been referred to antenatal clinic by her community midwife. She has a breech presentation confirmed on ultrasound scan so you refer her for ECV, but unfortunately this is not successful. You counsel the patient about the risks of elective Caesarean section at 39 weeks gestation compared with planned vaginal breech delivery. What is the risk of perinatal mortality with an elective Caesarean section?

Options for questions 36 - 37

A. Low dose aspirin

B. Low dose aspirin and LMWH prophylaxis

C. Thromboprophylaxis

D. Folic acid 5 g

E. Folic acid 400 mg

F. Transfuse 2-3 units RBC until Hb 100 g/l, then top up in a week until Hb 120-130 g/l

G. Aim for top up of 2 RBC units at 37-38 weeks

H. Aim for top up of 2 RBC units at 39-40 weeks

I. Chelation therapy p.o.

J. Chelation therapy i.v.

K. Chelation therapy s.c

L. Desferrioxamine 2g/24 hrs i.v

M. Liver MRI

N. Refer to surgeons

O. USS for viability

P. Wait and see

Obstetrics paper 2 – Questions

Instructions

For each clinical scenario below, choose the single most appropriate management option from the list. Each option maybe used once, more than once, or not at all.

36. A G2P1 (SVDX1) at 18+4 weeks gestation with a BMI of 29 is known to have β-thalassaemia major. She had a myocardial infarction 2 years ago and a recent ECHO has shown a low ejection fraction. She had 2 units RBC transfused 2 weeks ago and her recent Hb is 106 g/l, PLTS 468 x 109/L.

37. A G2P1 (SVDX1) at 12+2 weeks gestation with a BMI of 28 is known to have β-thalassaemia major. She has retained her spleen. Her liver iron is 18 mg/g (dw). She had 2 units RBC transfused 2 weeks ago and her Hb now is 106 g/l, PLTS 452 x 109/L.

Options for questions 38 - 40

    A. Stillbirth
    B. Neonatal death
    C. Late foetal loss
    D. Extended perinatal death
    E. Maternal death
    F. Maternity
    G. Ectopic pregnancy
    H. Early foetal loss
    I. Maternal mortality ratio
    J. Late maternal death
    K. Direct maternal death
    L. Indirect maternal death
    M. Maternal mortality rate
    N. Coincidental death during pregnancy

Instructions

Select the most appropriate classification from the list above.
Each option maybe used once, more than once, or not at all.

38. All stillbirths and neonatal deaths as reported by MBRRACE-UK.

39. The death of a woman while pregnant or within 42 days of termination of pregnancy, irrespective of the duration and site of the pregnancy, from any cause related to or aggravated by the pregnancy or its management but not from accidental or incidental causes.

40. Maternal deaths per 100,000 live births.

Options for questions 41 - 43

A. 2-5 in 1000 procedures in 10 years
B. Up to 15% of bowel injuries might not be diagnosed at the time of surgery
C. 1 in 10
D. 1 in 20
E. 4 in 100
F. 9 in 100
G. 11 in 100
H. 21 in 100
I. 3-6 in 1000
J. 1 in 2000

Instructions

When obtaining consent for an obstetric procedure, outline the operative risk that you would quote to the patient in each clinical scenario below. Each option maybe used once, more than once, or not at all.

41. The risk of facial or scalp lacerations of foetus following instrumental delivery.

42. The risk of foetal subgaleal haematoma at instrumental delivery.

43. The risk of perineal pain and dyspareunia after 3rd degree tear repair.

Options for questions 44 - 47

A. Immediately
B. 3 days
C. 5 days
D. 7 days
E. 10 days
F. 2 weeks
G. 3 weeks
H. 4 weeks
I. 6 weeks
J. 3 months
K. 4 months
L. 6 months
M. 12 months
N. No need
O. At the time of mifepristone administration
P. At the time of misoprostol administration
Q. After the uterine cavity has been emptied

Obstetrics paper 2 – Questions

Instructions

For each clinical scenario below, choose the single most appropriate option from the list. Each option maybe used once, more than once, or not at all.

44. A 29-year-old woman who had unprotected intercourse 25 days after normal vaginal delivery has been given ulipristal acetate for emergency contraception. She is breastfeeding. How long does she need to express and discard milk for before it is safe to breastfeed again?

45. A 24-year-old woman had an elective C-section for breech presentation today. She is planning to breastfeed for at least 6 months. She got on well with her combined contraceptive pill and would like to know when it is safe to start taking it again for contraceptive purposes. What would you advise her?

46. A 27-year-old woman who had a Caesarean section 4 days ago would like a Mirena coil fitted as soon as possible. When can she have one inserted?

47. A 21-year-old woman is having a medical termination of pregnancy at 10+6 weeks gestation. She lives a long way from health care services so would like to have a progesterone-only implant inserted at the earliest opportunity. When can this be done?

Options for questions 48 - 50

    A. Stillbirth

    B. Neonatal death

    C. Late foetal loss

    D. Extended perinatal death

    E. Maternal death

    F. Maternity

    G. Ectopic pregnancy

    H. Early foetal loss

    I. Maternal mortality ratio

    J. Late maternal death

    K. Direct maternal death

    L. Indirect maternal death

    M. Maternal mortality rate

    N. Coincidental death during pregnancy

Instructions

For each clinical scenario below, select the most appropriate classification from the list. Each option maybe used once, more than once, or not at all.

48. A 42-year-old lady who delivered a healthy child by Caesarean section unfortunately died 7 months later of cardiomyopathy.

49. A 39 week pregnant lady presented to A&E feeling unwell. She was diagnosed with genitourinary sepsis but was not given antibiotic treatment in a timely manner. She died 8 hours after admission.

50. A lady who was 33 weeks pregnant experienced headaches, which she had treated with Chinese herbal medicines. She was found dead the next morning and a post-mortem confirmed that the death was caused by the herbal medication she took.

Gynaecology paper 1 - Answers

1.B When treating women with PMS, drospirenone-containing COCs may represent effective treatment for PMS and should be considered as a first-line pharmaceutical intervention. There is emerging data which suggests use of the contraceptive pill continuously rather than cyclically.

2.C Use of a percutaneous (topical) oestradiol treatment is indicated due to previous DVT eg. oestradiol patch; however endometrial protection is required through use of a cyclical micronized progesterone (10–12 day course, either oral or vaginal progesterone) or a long-term progestogen with the LNG-IUS 52 mg .

Reference:
RCOG Green-Top Guideline No. 48: Management of premenstrual syndrome, November 2016.

3.P Offer vaginal oestrogen (pessary) for the treatment of OAB symptoms in postmenopausal women with vaginal atrophy.

4.M Mirabegron is recommended as an option for treating the symptoms of overactive bladder only for people in whom antimuscarinic drugs are contraindicated or clinically ineffective, or have unacceptable side effects.

5.J Do not use duloxetine as a first-line treatment for women with predominant stress UI. Do not routinely offer duloxetine as a second-line treatment for women with stress UI, although it may be offered as second-line therapy if women prefer pharmacological to surgical treatment, or are not suitable for surgical treatment. If duloxetine is prescribed, counsel women about its adverse effects.

6.N Offer one of the following choices first to women with OAB or mixed UI: oxybutynin (immediate release), or tolterodine (immediate release), or darifenacin (once daily preparation). If the first treatment for OAB or mixed UI is not effective or well-tolerated, offer another drug with the lowest acquisition cost.

References:
NICE Guideline (CG171): Urinary incontinence in women: management, November 2015.

NICE Guideline: Mirabegron for treating symptoms of overactive bladder, June 2013.

7.E Ovarian torsion will often show peripherally arranged follicles in addition to ovarian enlargement and oedema. In ovarian torsion every effort should be made to save the ovary by untwisting it and draining any cysts. A consultant with the relevant expertise should be involved. Even if the ovary appears black and necrotic, in most cases it will usually recover and result in a functional ovary.

8.B Discharge, no further investigations are required: any cyst which is simple and less than 5cm does not require any follow up unless the child has not yet achieved menarche.

9.A As she is asymptomatic and this was an incidental finding an annual pelvic ultrasound scan follow up is advised.

In the non-acute setting if the child/young woman has achieved menarche then the following investigations apply:

Simple cyst <5 cm	Simple cyst 5-7 cm	Simple cyst > 7cm	Complex cyst
No further investigations required	Annual USS follow-up	Consider MRI (or surgery)	LDH, bHCG, AFP, Ca125 Discuss further imaging with radiology

In any child who has not achieved menarche, further follow-up will be required for a cyst of any size.

Reference:
BritSPAG: Guideline for the management of ovarian cysts in children and adolescents, June 2017

10.B Up to 15% of bowel injuries may not be diagnosed at the time of surgery.

11.E A 4:100 risk of serious complications from abdominal hysterectomy.

12.A 2-5:1000 procedures in 10 years.

References:
Diagnostic laparoscopy,
RCOG Consent advice no.2, June 2017

Abdominal hysterectomy for benign conditions,
RCOG Consent advice no. 4, May 2009

Female sterilisation,
RCOG Consent advice no.3, February 2016

Laparoscopic management of tubal ectopic pregnancy,
RCOG Consent advice no.8, June 2010

Surgical evacuation of the uterus for early pregnancy loss,
RCOG Consent advice no. 10, June 2010

13. H Mayer Rokitansky Küster Hauser (MRKH)

14. A Complete androgen insensitivity syndrome

15. J Swyer syndrome

	MRKH	CAIS	SWYER	TURNER
Chromosomes	46 XX	46XY	46XY	45XO
Vagina	Dimple	Blind ending	Yes	Yes
Uterus	No	No	Yes	Yes
Axillary hair	Yes	Yes	No	No
Breasts	Yes	No	No	No
Gonads	Yes	Streak	Streak	Yes

Reference:
Garden, Hernon, Topping Paediatric and Adolescent Gynaecology for the MRCOG and Beyond, 2nd edition, August 2008

16.B EC providers should advise women that the Cu-IUD is the most effective method of emergency contraception.

Gynaecology paper 1 – Answers

17.L Ulipristal acetate EC (UPA-EC) has been demonstrated to be effective for EC up to 120 hours after UPSI.

18.G Levonorgestrel EC (LNG-EC) is licensed for EC up to 72 hours after UPSI.

19.G Evidence suggests that LNG-EC is ineffective if taken more than 96 hours after UPSI.

20.B Effectiveness of the Cu-IUD is not known to be affected by weight or BMI

References:
FSRH Guideline: Emergency contraception; updated May 2017

FSRH Guideline: UK medical eligibility criteria; 2016

21.E Less than 5% of endometrial hyperplasia without atypia will progress to endometrial carcinoma over 20 years.

22. F The minimum duration of oral progestogens for the treatment of endometrial hyperplasia without atypia is 6 months in order to induce histological regression.

23.J Hysterectomy is indicated where there is no histological regression of hyperplasia (without atypia) following 12 months of treatment.

Reference:
RCOG Green-Top Guideline No. 67: Management of endometrial hyperplasia, February 2016

24. F Lichen sclerosus - the symptoms include: itch, soreness, dyspareunia (if introital narrowing) and urinary symptoms. Signs include: pale, white areas; purpura (echymosis); fissuring; erosions; hyperkeratosis; localized or figure-8 distribution with loss of vulval architecture (resorption of labia minora, labial fusion, buried clitoris)

25. L Vulval psoriasis, which usually presents with well demarcated, glossy erythematous plaques. It lacks scale (in the vulva and flexures) due to friction rapidly rubbing away the scaly surface plaque; however silver grey scale may be evident if plaques extend down the thighs or on other skin surfaces.

Reference:
BASHH.UK national guideline on the management of vulval conditions. February 2014

26. B Urogenital symptoms (vaginal dryness) are the key symptom, hence a titrated dose of vaginal oestrogen would be the most appropriate first line treatment. A long term treatment regimen carries minimal risk. A vaginal cream, tablet or ring treatment would be suitable, but where there is dyspareunia, a cream/tablet pessary form may be more acceptable for the patient.

27. I This was a provoked DVT following an operative procedure; however the lowest risk VTE option is with transdermal oestrogen, which confers no greater than the general population risk with a Mirena IUS for endometrial protection.

28. G This was a provoked DVT following an operative procedure; however the lowest risk VTE option is with transdermal oestrogen which confers no greater than the general population risk. Unopposed oestrogen can be given as she does not have a uterus.

Reference:
NICE Guideline No 23. Menopause: diagnosis and management. November 2015.

Gynaecology paper 1 – Answers

29. **L** Where the combined oral contraceptive pill is contraindicated (eg. high BMI, VTE, migraine) spironolactone is a weak diuretic with anti-androgenic properties. It can be prescribed at 25-100mg daily.

30. **M** Yasmin is a combined oral contraceptive pill containing drosperinone, a derivative of spironolactone, which has antiandrogenic properties.

31. **H** Chronic anovulation and obesity brings a risk of endometrial hyperplasia and adenocarcinoma, hence a Mirena IUS is an alternative treatment where cyclical hormonal therapy is not optimal.

Reference:
Balen AH. Polycystic ovary syndrome (PCOS). The Obstetrician & Gynaecologist 2017;19:119 – 29. DOI:10.1111/tog.12345

32. **B** Bladder pain syndrome is a diagnosis of exclusion. All other investigations have been normal.

Reference:
RCOG Green-Top Guideline No. 70: Management of bladder pain syndrome, December 2016

33. **G** She has not had urodynamic studies, hence a diagnosis of urodynamic stress incontinence cannot be made. She has urinary urgency and increased frequency which is suggestive of OAB, and she also describes urinary incontinence after coughing, which may be due to cough-induced detrusor overactivity.

Reference:
NICE guideline CG171 : Urinary incontinence in women; September 2013, last updated 2015.

34. G All women with Y chromosome should have gonadectomy to prevent malignant transformation.

35. C Perform blood test for 21 OH – Ab and TPO – Ab as recommended for all women with suspected immune disorders. In view of asthma, hay fever and dermatitis she could potentially have other auto-immune disorders that have not yet been diagnosed.

Reference:
ESHRE Guideline: Management of women with premature ovarian insufficiency, December 2015

36. O She reported menorrhagia with hirsutism and required reliable contraception so the drospirenone-containing COCP would give an anti-androgen effect and improve menorrhagia. Mirena IUS would be an alternative option but is unlikely to improve hirsutism.

37. N A vaginal hysterectomy would be appropriate in this case as she has previously tried hormonal treatments including the Mirena IUS. Endometrial ablation was not effective and she has recurrent CIN3 which will need treatment. Colposcopy at the beginning of the procedure will aid complete resection.

38. N A vaginal hysterectomy would be appropriate in this case as she has previously undergone endometrial ablation which was not effective and hormonal treatments are likely to be contraindicated (dependent on her breast cancer receptor status.) Tamoxifen incurs an increased risk of endometrial carcinoma (1:500 chance.)

Reference:
NICE Guideline CG88: Heavy menstrual bleeding: assessment and management 2018.

39.M UAE is a highly effective treatment option with 80-90% of patients becoming asymptomatic or having significantly improved symptoms after one year. Fibroid volume is reduced by 40-70% and hysterectomy maybe required in up to 2.9% of cases.

References:
RCOG: Clinical recommendations on the use of UAE in the management of fibroids, 2013.

NICE Guideline CG88: Heavy menstrual bleeding: assessment and management 2018.

40.I TXA is a non-hormonal treatment for menorrhagia which can be used as an alternative to hormonal treatments.

Reference:
As above

41.G Intravesical lidocaine is a local anaesthetic which acts by blocking sensory nerve fibres within the bladder. Intravesical resiniferatoxin and bacillus Calmette-Guerin are not recommended treatments.

42.A Amitriptyline or cimetidine maybe considered when conservative measures have proved ineffective. Titration of the dose of amitriptyline from 10mg-100mg have shown improvement in pain scores when compared to untreated patients. Cimetidine should only be prescribed by a specialist clinician with experience in managing BPS as it is not licenced.

43.K This patient is keen to avoid any operative procedures so PTNS would be a suitable alternative following a multidisciplinary review.

Reference:
RCOG Green-Top Guideline No 70: Management of bladder pain syndrome December 2016

44. G When low-grade dyskaryosis is reported on a cytology sample, an automatic HR-HPV test will be performed. If the HR-HPV test is positive, the woman should be referred for colposcopy. If the HR-HPV test is negative, the woman should be returned to routine recall. Treatment at first visit to colposcopy for a referral of borderline or low-grade dyskaryosis should not be offered.

45. F In cases in which the source of the abnormal glandular cells is likely to be the endometrium or another gynaecological site, the woman should be referred to a gynaecology clinic. If a woman is not referred directly, the GP must make an urgent referral through the 'two-week wait' pathway.

46. I The significance of cytologically benign endometrial cells in cervical samples varies with the phase of the menstrual cycle, medication prescribed, clinical history and age of the woman; however in a population-based cervical screening programme, often this information is not available.

In women over the age of 40, normal endometrial cells are significantly more likely to be found in the cervical sample up to the 12th day of the menstrual cycle than in the remainder of the cycle, and need not be specifically reported by the laboratory. In women aged over 40, who are beyond the 12th day of the menstrual cycle, the finding of normal endometrial cells in a cervical sample may indicate endometrial pathology ranging from benign polyps to carcinoma. The association of normal endometrial cells in a cervical sample with significant pathology (endometrial hyperplasia and neoplasia) increases with age: it has been reported that endometrial disease may be found in up to 13% of women over the age of 60 with normal endometrial cells in their sample. However, normal endometrial cells found beyond the 12th day of the menstrual cycle in an individual over 40 may not indicate pathology if the woman is taking oral contraceptives, hormone replacement therapy, or tamoxifen, or where an IUCD has been fitted.

47. A After three consecutive inadequate samples a woman should be referred to colposcopy. She should be seen by the colposcopist within six weeks of referral.

48. N Unscheduled cervical screening does not form part of the NHSCSP. Provided a woman has undergone screening within the recommended interval (depending on her age), she should not be re-screened:

- on taking, or starting to take, an oral contraceptive
- on insertion of an intrauterine contraceptive device (IUD)
- on taking or starting to take hormone replacement therapy (HRT)
- in association with pregnancy (antenatally or postnatally)
- on being diagnosed with genital warts or pelvic infection
- due to heavy cigarette smoking
- due to having multiple sexual partners

Women with cervical symptoms, including persistent vaginal discharge that cannot be otherwise explained (eg by an infection), should be referred in a timely manner for further evaluation of the cervix. The indications for performing cervical cytology in GUM clinics are no different to those for the rest of the NHSCSP. Cervical samples taken for screening purposes in GUM clinics should be restricted to women who have not been screened in the previous routine screening interval, with the exception of HIV positive women.

Reference:
NHS Cervical Screening Programme: Colposcopy and programme management, Third Edition, March 2016

49. A

50. B In pregnancies <12 weeks gestation, anti-D Ig prophylaxis is only indicated following ectopic pregnancy, molar pregnancy, therapeutic termination of pregnancy and in cases of uterine bleeding where this is repeated, heavy or associated with abdominal pain. The minimum dose should be 250 IU. A test for feto-maternal haemorrhage (FMH) is not required.

Reference:
BCSH Guideline for the use of anti-D immunoglobulin for the prevention of haemolytic disease of the foetus and newborn, 2014

Obstetric paper 1 - Answers

1. C

2. A

3. C

Reference:
NICE Guideline: Hypertension in pregnancy: Diagnosis and management; January 2011

4. **E** Women with persistent pruritus and normal biochemistry should have LFTs repeated every 1–2 weeks.

5. **B** Obstetric cholestasis is diagnosed when otherwise unexplained pruritus occurs in pregnancy where abnormal LFTs and/or raised BA occur in the pregnant woman and both resolve after delivery.

6. **D** Women should be advised that where the prothrombin time is prolonged, the use of water-soluble vitamin K (menadiol sodium phosphate) in doses of 5–10 mg daily is indicated. Women should be advised that when prothrombin time is normal, water-soluble vitamin K (menadiol sodium phosphate) in low doses should be used only after careful counselling about the likely benefits but small theoretical risk.

Reference:
RCOG Green-Top Guideline No. 43: Obstetric cholestasis, April 2011

7. A Mild pain may be managed in the community with rest, oral fluids and paracetamol or weak opioids. NSAIDs should be used only between 12 and 28 weeks of gestation. Primary care physicians should have a low threshold for referring women to secondary care; all women with pain which does not settle with simple analgesia, who are febrile, have atypical pain or chest pain or symptoms of shortness of breath, should be referred to hospital.

8. C Acute stroke, both ischaemic and haemorrhagic, is associated with SCD, and this diagnosis should be considered in any woman with SCD who presents with acute neurological impairment. Acute stroke is a medical emergency and a rapid-exchange blood transfusion can decrease long-term neurological damage. If a stroke is suspected, the woman should have urgent brain imaging and the on call haematologist should be consulted for consideration of urgent exchange transfusion. Thrombolysis is not indicated in acute stroke secondary to SCD.

References:
RCOG Green-Top Guideline No. 61: Management of sickle cell disease in pregnancy, July 2011.

British Society for Haematology. Management of acute chest syndrome in sickle cell disease. March 2015.

9. B Anti-D and anti-c levels should be measured every 4 weeks up to 28 weeks gestation and then every 2 weeks until delivery. The cause of the alloimmunisation should be ascertained: for example, inadequate or omitted anti-D prophylaxis or a previous blood transfusion. Details of previously affected pregnancies, particularly IUTs and the gestation at which they were commenced, neonatal anaemia, gestation at delivery and the need for exchange transfusions or phototherapy, should also be obtained. This information enables a risk assessment of the pregnancy to be made. Ultrasound monitoring should commence once there is a moderate or severe risk of foetal anaemia.

10.D The presence of anti-E potentiates the severity of foetal anaemia due to anti-c antibodies so referral at lower levels/titres is indicated (unless the foetus has only one of these antigens). IUT might not be necessary.

11.D For anti-K antibodies, referral should take place once detected, as severe foetal anaemia can occur even with low titres. Anti-K titres appear to correlate poorly with the severity of disease with foetal anaemia occurring at titres as low as 8.

Reference:
RCOG Green-Top Guideline No. 65: The management of women with red cell antibodies during pregnancy; May 2014.

12.A This lady has already had red cells and FFP hence cryoprecipitate is now required at a standard dose of two 5-unit pools. Subsequent cryoprecipitate transfusion should be guided by fibrinogen results, aiming to keep levels above 1.5 g/l.

FFP at a dose of 12–15 ml/kg should be administered for every 6 units of red cells during major obstetric haemorrhage. Subsequent FFP transfusion should be guided by the results of clotting tests if they are available in a timely manner, aiming to maintain prothrombin time (PT) and activated partial thromboplastin time (APTT) ratios at less than 1.5 x normal.

The FFP and cryoprecipitate should ideally be of the same group as the recipient. If unavailable, FFP of a different ABO group is acceptable provided that it does not have a high titre of anti-A or anti-B activity. No anti-D prophylaxis is required if a RhD-negative woman receives RhD-positive FFP or cryoprecipitate.

13. J Aim to maintain the platelet count above 50 x 10^9/l in the acutely bleeding patient.

A platelet transfusion trigger of 75 x 10^9/l is recommended to provide a margin of safety.

The platelets should ideally be group compatible. RhD-negative women should also receive RhD-negative platelets.

Reference:
RCOG Green-Top Guideline No. 47: Transfusion in obstetrics, May 2015.

14. B Women with thalassaemia who have undergone splenectomy and have a platelet count above 600 x 10^9/l should be offered low-molecular-weight heparin thromboprophylaxis as well as low-dose aspirin (75 mg/day.)

15. C Women with thalassaemia who are not already using prophylactic low-molecular-weight heparin should be advised to use it during antenatal hospital admissions.

16. G The decision to initiate a transfusion regimen is a clinical one based on the woman's symptoms and foetal growth. If the haemoglobin is less than 80 g/l then aim for a top-up transfusion of 2 units at 37–38 weeks of gestation. Generally, in non-transfused patients, if the haemoglobin is above 80 g/l at 36 weeks of gestation, transfusion can be avoided prior to delivery. Postnatal transfusion can be provided as necessary.

Reference:
RCOG Green-top guideline No. 66: Management of beta thalassaemia in pregnancy, March 2014.

17. G The choice of contraceptive method should be initiated by 21 days after childbirth.

18. **A** Women should be advised that intrauterine contraception (IUC) and progestogen-only implant (IMP) can be inserted immediately after delivery.

19. **A** As above.

20. **H** Oral EC levonorgestrel 1.5 mg (LNG-EC) and ulipristal acetate 30 mg (UPA-EC) are safe to use from 21 days after childbirth. The copper intrauterine device (Cu-IUD) is safe to use for EC from 28 days after childbirth.

Reference:
FSRH Guideline: Contraception after pregnancy, January 2017.

21. **D** In the event of continual uterine bleeding which is clinically judged to represent the same sensitising event, with no features suggestive of a new presentation or a significant change in the pattern or severity of bleeding, such as the presence of abdominal pain or another clinical presentation. A minimum dose of 500 IU anti-D Ig should be given at six weekly intervals. In the event of further intermittent uterine bleeding, estimation of FMH should be carried out at two weekly intervals. In this situation non-invasive foetal RHD typing using maternal plasma could be considered to reduce hospital attendance, blood sampling and avoid repeated administration of doses of anti-D, balanced against the small risk of false negativity (0·08–0·16%, Clausen et al., 2002; Finning et al., 2008) of foetal D typing by this technique. If the two weekly FMH test shows the presence of foetal cells, additional anti-D Ig should be administered to cover the volume of FMH. The additional dose should be calculated as 125 IU if administered IM or 100 IU if administered IV for each mL of foetal red cells detected (minimum 500IU).

22. **F** For potentially sensitising events after 20 weeks gestation, a minimum anti-D Ig dose of 500 IU should be administered within 72 hours of the event. A test for FMH is required.

Reference:
BCSH Guideline for the use of anti-D immunoglobulin for the prevention of haemolytic disease of the foetus and newborn, 2014

23. I Vicryl 3.0 (polyglactin) should be used to repair the anorectal mucosa as it may cause less irritation and discomfort than polydioxanone (PDS) sutures.

Reference:
RCOG Green-top Guideline No. 29: The management of third and fourth degree perineal tears, June 2015.

24. N Mersilene tape with double-ended needles will provide ease of use with a non-absorbable material.

Reference:
Gibb D, Saridogan E. The role of transabdominal cervical cerclage techniques in maternity care. The Obstetrician & Gynaecologist 2016;18: 117–25. DOI: 10.1111/tog.12254.

25. F Vicryl size 1 suture on a curved 70mm needle gives an adequate length of needle to place the uterine brace suture accurately.

Reference:
ALSG MOET Course Skill E4 B-Lynch brace handout sheet. Last updated 13/02/2014.

26. A When repair of the EAS and/or IAS muscle is being performed, either monofilament sutures such as 3-0 PDS or modern braided sutures such as 2-0 polyglactin can be used with equivalent outcomes.

Reference:
RCOG Green-Top Guideline No. 29: The management of third and fourth degree perineal tears, June 2015.

Obstetric paper 1 – Answers

27. G Where a woman presents with an unplanned vaginal breech labour, management should depend on the stage of labour, whether factors associated with increased complications are found, availability of appropriate clinical expertise and informed consent. Women near or in active second stage of labour should not be routinely offered Caesarean section. Where time and circumstances permit, the position of the foetal neck and legs and the foetal weight should be estimated using ultrasound, and the woman counselled about a planned vaginal breech birth. All maternity units must be able to provide skilled supervision for vaginal breech birth where a woman is admitted in advanced labour and protocols for this eventuality should be developed.

28. M Women should be informed that a higher risk planned vaginal breech birth is expected where there are independent indications for Caesarean section and in the following circumstances:

- Hyperextended neck on ultrasound.
- High estimated foetal weight (more than 3.8 kg).
- Low estimated weight (less than tenth centile).
- Footling presentation.
- Evidence of antenatal foetal compromise.

The role of pelvimetry is unclear.

29. O The presence of a skilled birth attendant is essential for safe vaginal breech birth.

Reference:
RCOG Green-Top Guideline No. 20b: Management of breech presentation; March 2017

30.H Following a potentially sensitising event (including ECV,) anti-D Ig should be administered as soon as possible but always aiming for treatment within 72 hours of the event.

31.H Following a potentially sensitising event (including RTA,) anti-D Ig should be administered as soon as possible but always aiming for treatment within 72 hours of the event.

Reference:
BCSH guideline for the use of anti-D immunoglobulin for the prevention of haemolytic disease of the foetus and newborn, January 2014.

Please refer to the Anti-D checklist on page 136

32.D Explain to the patient that the likelihood of maternal GBS carriage in this pregnancy is 50%. Discuss the options of IAP, or bacteriological testing in late pregnancy, and then offer IAP if still positive. If performed, bacteriological testing should ideally be carried out at 35–37 weeks of gestation or 3–5 weeks prior to the anticipated delivery date, e.g. 32–34 weeks of gestation for women with twins.

33.H IAP should be offered to women with a previous baby with early- or late-onset GBS disease.

Obstetric paper 1 – Answers

34.A A maternal request is not an indication for bacteriological screening. When testing for GBS carrier status, a swab should be taken from the lower vagina and the anorectum. A single swab (vagina then anorectum) or two different swabs can be used.

35.K Clinicians should offer IAP to women with GBS bacteriuria identified during the current pregnancy. Women with GBS urinary tract infection (growth >105 cfu/ml) during pregnancy should receive appropriate treatment at the time of diagnosis as well as IAP.

Reference:
RCOG Guideline No. 36: Prevention of early onset neonatal group B streptococcal disease, September 2017

36.O Antenatal risk factors for this lady: age, parity, smoker and immobility – hence she requires prophylaxis both antenatally and until she is 6 weeks postnatal. The correct treatment given her weight would be enoxaparin 60mg once daily.

37.G Antenatal risk factors for this lady: OHSS + IVF pregnancy – hence she needs antenatal prophylaxis (particularly for the first trimester risk seen in OHSS.) The correct antenatal dose for her weight would be 5000iu dalteparin once daily but we don't currently know what her postnatal risk factors will be.

38.J Antenatal risk factors for this lady: hospital admission and IBD. These factors are both in the intermediate risk group and therefore she would require antenatal prophylaxis. Postnatally the IBD would give an ongoing risk factor as well as being on antenatal LMWH hence treatment for 6 weeks following delivery should be offered. The correct dose for her weight would be 5000iu dalteparin once daily.

39.O Antenatal risk factors for this lady: BMI 30+, IBD, varicose veins. She scores 4+ in the risk assessment chart and hence needs antenatal prophylaxis. These risk factors would be maintained postnatally hence continuing for 6 weeks following delivery should be discussed. The correct dose for her weight would be 60mg enoxaparin once daily.

40.G Antenatal risk factors for this lady: infection and vomiting, hospital admission. She needs prophylaxis for the period of hospital admission with the correct dose for her weight being 5000iu dalteparin once daily.

References:
To view the summary of risk factors please see the following flow charts taken from the RCOG Thromboembolic Disorders Guidelines

RCOG Green-Top Guideline No 37a: Reducing the risk of venous thromboembolism during pregnancy and the puerperium, April 2015

RCOG Green-Top Guideline No 37b: Thromboembolic disease in pregnancy and the puerperium; acute management, April 2015

Appendix I: Obstetric thromboprophylaxis risk assessment and management

Antenatal assessment and management (to be assessed at booking and repeated if admitted)

Any previous VTE except a single event related to major surgery

➡ **HIGH RISK**
Requires antenatal prophylaxis with LMWH
Refer to trust-nominated thrombosis in pregnancy expert/team

- Hospital admission
- Single previous VTE related to major surgery
- High-risk thrombophilia + no VTE
- Medical comorbidities e.g. cancer, heart failure, active SLE, IBD or inflammatory polyarthropathy, nephrotic syndrome, type I DM with nephropathy, sickle cell disease, current IVDU
- Any surgical procedure e.g. appendicectomy
- OHSS (first trimester only)

➡ **INTERMEDIATE RISK**
Consider antenatal prophylaxis with LMWH

- Obesity (BMI > 30 kg/m²)
- Age > 35
- Parity ≥ 3
- Smoker
- Gross varicose veins
- Current pre-eclampsia
- Immobility, e.g. paraplegia, PGP
- Family history of unprovoked or estrogen-provoked VTE in first-degree relative
- Low-risk thrombophilia
- Multiple pregnancy
- IVF/ART
- Transient risk factors: Dehydration/hyperemesis; current systemic infection; long-distance travel

4
➡ **Four or more risk factors: prophylaxis from first trimester**

3
Three risk factors: prophylaxis from 28 weeks

Fewer than three risk factors

➡ **LOWER RISK**
Mobilisation and avoidance of dehydration

Postnatal assessment and management (to be assessed on delivery suite)

Any previous VTE
Anyone requiring antenatal LMWH
High-risk thrombophilia
Low-risk thrombophilia + FHx

→ **HIGH RISK** — At least 6 weeks' postnatal prophylactic LMWH

Caesarean section in labour
BMI ≥ 40 kg/m²
Readmission or prolonged admission (≥ 3 days) in the puerperium
Any surgical procedure in the puerperium except immediate repair of the perineum
Medical comorbidities e.g. cancer, heart failure, active SLE, IBD or inflammatory polyarthropathy; nephrotic syndrome, type I DM with nephropathy, sickle cell disease, current IVDU

→ **INTERMEDIATE RISK** — At least 10 days' postnatal prophylactic LMWH

NB If persisting or > 3 risk factors consider extending thromboprophylaxis with LMWH

Age > 35 years
Obesity (BMI ≥ 30 kg/m²)
Parity ≥ 3
Smoker
Elective caesarean section
Family history of VTE
Low-risk thrombophilia
Gross varicose veins
Current systemic infection
Immobility, e.g. paraplegia, PGP, long-distance travel
Current pre-eclampsia
Multiple pregnancy
Preterm delivery in this pregnancy (< 37⁺⁰ weeks)
Stillbirth in this pregnancy
Mid-cavity rotational or operative delivery
Prolonged labour (> 24 hours)
PPH > 1 litre or blood transfusion

Two or more risk factors → (INTERMEDIATE RISK)

Fewer than two risk factors → **LOWER RISK** — Early mobilisation and avoidance of dehydration

Antenatal and postnatal prophylactic dose of LMWH
Weight < 50 kg = 20 mg enoxaparin/2500 units dalteparin/3500 units tinzaparin daily
Weight 50–90 kg = 40 mg enoxaparin/5000 units dalteparin/4500 units tinzaparin daily
Weight 91–130 kg = 60 mg enoxaparin/7500 units dalteparin/7000 units tinzaparin daily
Weight 131–170 kg = 80 mg enoxaparin/10000 units dalteparin/9000 units tinzaparin daily
Weight > 170 kg = 0.6 mg/kg/day enoxaparin/ 75 u/kg/day dalteparin/ 75 u/kg/day tinzaparin

Obstetric paper 1 – Answers

Appendix III: Risk assessment for venous thromboembolism (VTE)

- If total score ≥ 4 antenatally, consider thromboprophylaxis from the first trimester.
- If total score 3 antenatally, consider thromboprophylaxis from 28 weeks.
- If total score ≥ 2 postnatally, consider thromboprophylaxis for at least 10 days.
- If admitted to hospital antenatally consider thromboprophylaxis.
- If prolonged admission (≥ 3 days) or readmission to hospital within the puerperium consider thromboprophylaxis.

For patients with an identified bleeding risk, the balance of risks of bleeding and thrombosis should be discussed in consultation with a haematologist with expertise in thrombosis and bleeding in pregnancy.

Risk factors for VTE

Pre-existing risk factors	Tick	Score
Previous VTE (except a single event related to major surgery)		4
Previous VTE provoked by major surgery		3
Known high-risk thrombophilia		3
Medical comorbidities e.g. cancer, heart failure; active systemic lupus erythematosus, inflammatory polyarthropathy or inflammatory bowel disease; nephrotic syndrome; type I diabetes mellitus with nephropathy; sickle cell disease; current intravenous drug user		3
Family history of unprovoked or estrogen-related VTE in first-degree relative		1
Known low-risk thrombophilia (no VTE)		1[a]
Age (> 35 years)		1
Obesity		1 or 2[b]
Parity ≥ 3		1
Smoker		1
Gross varicose veins		1
Obstetric risk factors		
Pre-eclampsia in current pregnancy		1
ART/IVF (antenatal only)		1
Multiple pregnancy		1
Caesarean section in labour		2
Elective caesarean section		1
Mid-cavity or rotational operative delivery		1
Prolonged labour (> 24 hours)		1
PPH (> 1 litre or transfusion)		1
Preterm birth < 37+0 weeks in current pregnancy		1
Stillbirth in current pregnancy		1
Transient risk factors		
Any surgical procedure in pregnancy or puerperium except immediate repair of the perineum, e.g. appendicectomy, postpartum sterilisation		3
Hyperemesis		3
OHSS (first trimester only)		4
Current systemic infection		1
Immobility, dehydration		1
TOTAL		

Abbreviations: ART assisted reproductive technology; IVF in vitro fertilisation; OHSS ovarian hyperstimulation syndrome; VTE venous thromboembolism.

[a] If the known low-risk thrombophilia is in a woman with a family history of VTE in a first-degree relative postpartum thromboprophylaxis should be continued for 6 weeks.

[b] BMI ≥ 30 = 1; BMI ≥ 40 = 2

Appendix IV: Summary of guideline for thromboprophylaxis in women with previous VTE and/or thrombophilia (also see Appendix I)

Very high risk	Previous VTE on long-term oral anticoagulant therapy	Recommend antenatal high-dose LMWH and at least 6 weeks' postnatal LMWH or until switched back to oral anticoagulant therapy
	Antithrombin deficiency Antiphospholipid syndrome with previous VTE	*These women require specialist management by experts in haemostasis and pregnancy*
High risk	Any previous VTE (except a single VTE related to major surgery)	Recommend antenatal and 6 weeks' postnatal prophylactic LMWH
Intermediate risk	Asymptomatic high-risk thrombophilia homozygous factor V Leiden/compound heterozygote Protein C or S deficiency	Refer to local expert Consider antenatal LMWH Recommend postnatal prophylactic LMWH for 6 weeks
	Single previous VTE associated with major surgery without thrombophilia, family history or other risk factors	Consider antenatal LMWH (but not routinely recommended) Recommend LMWH from 28 weeks of gestation and 6 weeks' postnatal prophylactic LMWH
Low risk	Asymptomatic low-risk thrombophilia (prothrombin gene mutation or factor V Leiden)	Consider as a risk factor and score appropriately (see Appendix III) Recommend 10 days' if other risk factor postpartum (or 6 weeks' if significant family history) postnatal prophylactic LMWH

41. A A stillbirth is the death of a baby occurring before or during birth once a pregnancy has reached 24 weeks.

42. B A neonatal death is a baby born alive at any time during the pregnancy, but dies within four weeks of being born.

43. C A baby born between 22 and 23 weeks of pregnancy, who shows no signs of life, regardless of when the baby died, is referred to as a late foetal loss (sometimes referred to as a late miscarriage).

ALL DEATHS (death during pregnancy, childbirth or puerperium		
MATERNAL DEATH		
Direct maternal death: • Abortive outcome • Hypertensive disorders • Obstetric haemorrhage • Pregnancy related infection • Other obstetric complications • Unanticipated complications	**Indirect maternal death:** • Non-obstetric complications	**Unknown Undetermined**

Coincidental category (these deaths occur in pregnancy, childbirth, or the puerperium but are not by definition considered maternal death)	Disease entity
	Motor vehicle accident
	External causes of accidental injury
	Assault
	Rape
	Event of undetermined intent
	Other accidents
	Herbal medication
	Other - specify

References:
MBRRACE-UK perinatal mortality surveillance report - UK perinatal deaths for 2015 births: Definitions page iii.

The WHO application of ICD-10 to deaths during pregnancy, childbirth and puerperium: ICD MM, WHO 2012.

International statistical classification of diseases and related health problems. – 10th revision, edition 2010.

44. G 11:100

45. C 1:10

References:
Caesarean section for placenta praevia, Consent advice no.12, December 2010

Operative vaginal delivery, Consent advice no.11, July 2010

Repair of third and fourth degree tears following childbirth, Consent advice no.9, June 2010

46. H Perform an USS for cervical length and offer a choice of either prophylactic vaginal progesterone or prophylactic cervical cerclage to women:

- with a history of spontaneous preterm birth or mid-trimester loss between 16+0 and 34+0 weeks of pregnancy and
- in whom a transvaginal ultrasound scan has been carried out between 16+0 and 24+0 weeks of pregnancy that reveals a cervical length of less than 25 mm.

Discuss the benefits and risks of prophylactic progesterone and cervical cerclage with the woman and take her preferences into account.

Reference:
NICE Guideline No 25: Preterm labour and birth, Nov 2015.

47.M The guideline recommends considering 'rescue' cervical cerclage for women between 16+0 and 27+6 weeks of pregnancy with a dilated cervix and exposed, unruptured foetal membranes: take into account gestational age (being aware that the benefits are likely to be greater for earlier gestations) and the extent of cervical dilatation; discuss with a consultant obstetrician and consultant paediatrician. In our case, however, the rescue cerclage is unsuitable as there is a foot protruding through the cervix which would pose a great risk of rupturing the membranes at the time of the procedure.

Reference:
As above.

48.H If the clinical assessment suggests that the woman is in suspected preterm labour and she is 30+0 weeks pregnant or more, consider a transvaginal ultrasound measurement of cervical length as a diagnostic test to determine the likelihood of birth within 48 hours.

Reference:
As above.

49. L Consider foetal fibronectin testing as a diagnostic test to determine the likelihood of birth within 48 hours for women who are 30+0 weeks pregnant or more if transvaginal ultrasound measurement of cervical length is indicated but is not available or not acceptable to the patient.

Reference:
As above.

50.C Pregnant women with antiphospholipid syndrome should be considered for treatment with low-dose aspirin plus heparin to prevent further miscarriage. The GTG states that antiphospholipid syndrome is defined as the association between antiphospholipid antibodies (lupus anticoagulant, anticardiolipin antibodies or anti-B2 glycoprotein-I antibodies) and either an adverse pregnancy outcome or vascular thrombosis. An adverse pregnancy outcome can be defined as:

- three or more consecutive miscarriages before 10 weeks of gestation

- one or more morphologically normal foetal losses after the 10th week of gestation

- one or more preterm births before the 34th week of gestation owing to placental disease (which is the case in this lady.)

- With a cervical excision depth of 8mm there does not appear to be an increased chance of prematurity as outlined by the meta-analysis by Kyrgiou et al. (2006.)

References:
Green-Top Guideline No 17: The investigation and treatment of couples with recurrent first trimester and second trimester miscarriage; April 2011.

Scientific Impact Paper no. 21: Reproductive outcomes after local treatment for pre-invasive cervical disease, July 2016.

Gynaecology paper 2 - Answers

1.N Unscheduled cervical screening does not form part of the NHSCSP. Provided a woman has undergone screening within the recommended interval (depending on her age), she should not be re-screened:

- on taking, or starting to take, an oral contraceptive
- on insertion of an intrauterine contraceptive device (IUD)
- on taking or starting to take hormone replacement therapy (HRT)
- in association with pregnancy (antenatally or postnatally)
- on being diagnosed with genital warts or pelvic infection
- due to heavy cigarette smoking
- due to having multiple sexual partners

Women with cervical symptoms, including persistent vaginal discharge that cannot be otherwise explained (eg by an infection), should be referred in a timely manner for further evaluation of the cervix. The indications for performing cervical cytology in GUM clinics are no different to those for the rest of the NHSCSP. Cervical samples taken for screening purposes in GUM clinics should be restricted to women who have not been screened in the previous routine screening interval, with the exception of HIV positive women.

2. N Women should be ceased from the programme where they do not have a cervix due to:

- having undergone total hysterectomy (women with a subtotal hysterectomy remain at risk and should remain in the programme)
- congenital absence of the cervix
- being a male-to-female transsexual
- having undergone a radical trachelectomy for cervical cancer

3. B Women must be referred for colposcopy after one test reported as high-grade dyskaryosis (moderate). A HR-HPV Test is not indicated/performed. Unless an excisional treatment is planned, biopsy should be carried out when the cytology indicates high-grade dyskaryosis (moderate) or worse and always when a recognisably atypical transformation zone is present. Cases occurring in pregnancy are an exception.

4. I Contact bleeding at the time of cervical sampling may occur, and is not an indication for referral to colposcopy in the absence of other symptoms and a normal smear result.

5. A All women exposed to DES in utero should have an initial colposcopic examination and where no abnormalities are found, they can be returned to routine screening. In cases where DES related cervical changes are found, annual colposcopy of the cervix and vagina should be undertaken.

Reference:
NHS Cervical screening programme: Colposcopy and programme management, 3rd edition March 2016

Gynaecology paper 2 – Answers

6. G LNG IUS is the first line pharmacological treatment option for HMB.

Reference:
NICE Guideline CG88: Heavy menstrual bleeding: assessment and management, 2018

7. G Where endometrial hyperplasia without atypia has been reported, a LNG IUS (or oral progestogens) should be offered.

8. G In light of her severe, poorly controlled COPD and morbid obesity she would have a significant risk of worsening morbidity/mortality following any form of anaesthetic required for a hysterectomy; hence LNG IUS (or oral progestogens) would be a lower risk strategy.

9. A Total abdominal hysterectomy and bilateral salpingo-oophorectomy is indicated where atypia has been reported and laparoscopic or vaginal approach would have a higher chance of failure/complication.

Reference:
RCOG Green Top Guideline No 67: Management of endometrial hyperplasia; February 2016

10. I PID is the most likely cause of her symptoms given her age, new partner and nature of pain with vaginal discharge.

11. C Diverticulitis is the most likely cause of her symptoms given her age, past medical and surgical history and she is not sexually active.

Reference:
Arulkumaran S, Symonds IM, Fowlie A. Oxford Handbook of Obstetrics and Gynaecology.(2005) Acute pelvic pain p564.

12. I Where there is a BMI>30 a transdermal oestrogen preparation should be offered with a progestogen treatment (ideally an IUS) for endometrial protection.

Reference:
NICE Guideline No 23. Menopause: Diagnosis and Management. November 2015.

13. O There is moderate evidence to support the use of CBT in anxiety and depression. The MENOS-1 study demonstrated the effectiveness of CBT for reducing the impact of hot flushes and night sweats in breast cancer patients.

Reference:
Mann E. at al. Lancet Oncology 2012; 13: 309-18.

14. E Continuous combined HRT, is likely to require a medium/high dose oestradiol. The alternative option is a combined oral contraceptive pill but bone mineralization and cardiovascular risk markers are more favourable in HRT users.

Reference:
Hillard, T, Abernethy K, Hamoda H, Shaw I, Everett M, Ayres J and Currie H. British Menopause Society. 2017. Management of the Menopause.

15. H Women requiring EC who are using enzyme-inducing drugs (such as St. John's wort) should be offered a Cu-IUD if appropriate. A 3 mg dose of LNG can be considered but women should be informed that the effectiveness of this regimen is unknown. A double-dose of UPA-EC is not recommended. If a woman is awaiting treatment for cervical cancer it is UKMEC 4 for Cu-IUD.

16. B EC providers should be aware that a Cu-IUD can be inserted up to 5 days after the first UPSI in a natural menstrual cycle, or up to 5 days after the earliest likely date of ovulation (whichever is later).

17. H Adolescents who need EC should be offered all methods of EC including the Cu-IUD, but given that she passed out following previous IUCD insertion, a Cu-IUD is a less acceptable option for her. If a Cu-IUD is not appropriate or not acceptable, women should be advised that oral EC should be taken as soon as possible if there has been UPSI within the last 5 days. Women should be informed that it is possible that higher weight or BMI could reduce the effectiveness of oral EC, particularly LNG-EC. In this particular case, a double dose of LNG EC is the best option since UPA EC maybe less effective as she has already had LNG EC within the past 7 days. Consider a double-dose (3 mg) LNG if BMI >26 or weight >70 kg or if taking an enzyme inducer.

18. G EC providers should be aware that the effectiveness of UPA-EC could theoretically be reduced if a woman has taken a progestogen in the 7 days prior to taking UPA-EC. UPA could also be less effective if a woman is taking an enzyme inducer.

19. C It is more than 5 days past her ovulation and hence oral EC is unlikely to work and IUD cannot be inserted as implantation could have already occurred. It's too early for a pregnancy test to be reliable.

References:
FSRH guideline: Emergency contraception; updated May 2017

FSRH guideline: UK Medical Eligibility Criteria; 2016

20. C Gonadotrophin therapy is indicated for women with anovulatory PCOS who have failed to ovulate with anti-oestrogens or if they have a response to clomifene that is likely to reduce their chance of conception eg persistently elevated LH levels.

21. D Ovarian drilling would be the best treatment option as she lives a long distance from the hospital and would be unable to attend for the intensive monitoring required for gonadotrophin therapy.

22. N None of the above. Recommend avoid sexual intercourse as high risk of multiple pregnancy and OHSS.

Reference:
Balen AH. Polycystic ovary syndrome (PCOS). The Obstetrician & Gynaecologist 2017;19:119 – 29. DOI:10.1111/tog.12345

23. F This lady has Turner's syndrome and therefore requires referral to a cardiologist, geneticist and endocrinologist for further investigation and management.

24. J All women diagnosed with POI on HRT require 5 yearly DEXA scans to assess bone density.

25. B Apart from other investigations for POI she needs Fragile X permutation test. The most common inherited cause of learning disability is Fragile X syndrome

Reference:
ESHRE guideline: Management of women with premature ovarian insufficiency, December 2015

Gynaecology paper 2 – Answers

26. J A 1:2000 failure rate following vasectomy.

27. E A 4-8:100 risk of persistent trophoblastic tissue with laparoscopic salpingotomy.

28. D A 1:20 risk of repeat surgical procedure following surgical evacuation of uterus.

References:
Diagnostic laparoscopy,
RCOG Consent advice no.2, June 1017

Abdominal hysterectomy for benign conditions,
RCOG Consent advice no. 4, May 2009

Female sterilisation,
RCOG Consent advice no.3, February 2016

Laparoscopic management of tubal ectopic pregnancy,
RCOG Consent advice no.8, June 2010

Surgical evacuation of the uterus for early pregnancy loss,
RCOG Consent advice no. 10, June 2010

29. K The use of desmopressin may be considered specifically to reduce nocturia in women with UI or OAB who find it a troublesome symptom. Use particular caution in women with cystic fibrosis and avoid in those over 65 years with cardiovascular disease or hypertension.

30. D After undertaking a detailed clinical history and examination, perform multi-channel filling and voiding cystometry before surgery in women who have: symptoms of OAB leading to a clinical suspicion of detrusor overactivity, or symptoms suggestive of voiding dysfunction or anterior compartment prolapse, or had previous surgery for stress incontinence. Consider ambulatory urodynamics or videourodynamics if the diagnosis is unclear after conventional urodynamics.

31. D As described this lady has possible OAB and moderate anterior vaginal wall prolapse. Therefore she should be referred for urodynamics as the guideline recommends this before surgery in women who have: symptoms of OAB leading to a clinical suspicion of detrusor overactivity, or symptoms suggestive of voiding dysfunction or anterior compartment prolapse, or had previous surgery for stress incontinence. Consider ambulatory urodynamics or videourodynamics if the diagnosis is unclear after conventional urodynamics.

32. H Offer percutaneous sacral nerve stimulation to women after MDT review if their OAB has not responded to conservative management including drugs, and they are unable to perform clean intermittent catheterisation.

References:
NICE guideline (CG171): Urinary incontinence in women: management, November 2015

NICE guideline: Mirabegron for treating symptoms of overactive bladder, June 2013

33. **F** A repeat biopsy should be performed following a minimum of 6 months of oral progestogen treatment.

34. **C** In women with atypical hyperplasia who do not undergo a hysterectomy endometrial surveillance (through endometrial biopsy) should be offered every three months until two consecutive negative biopsies are obtained.

Reference:
RCOG Green Top Guideline No. 67: Management of endometrial hyperplasia; February 2016

35. **H** Consider MRI (or surgery)

36. **L** Bloods: CA 125, LDH, bHGC, AFP

37. **C** Laparoscopy: Cysts that persist or increase in size are unlikely to be functional and may warrant surgical management and the patient should be referred to the paediatric and adolescent gynaecology clinic to decide upon further management. Any surgery on adolescents should be carried out by a gynaecologist with the appropriate laparoscopic surgical skills to reduce the need for an unnecessary laparotomy or oophorectomy. This is of great importance as having laparoscopic surgery as opposed to a laparotomy will reduce postoperative pain, length of hospital stay and reduce the chance of adhesions.

In the non-acute setting if the child/young woman has achieved menarche then the following investigations apply:

Simple cyst <5 cm	Simple cyst 5-7 cm	Simple cyst > 7cm	Complex cyst
No further investigations required	Annual USS follow-up	Consider MRI (or surgery)	LDH, bHCG, AFP, Ca125 Discuss further imaging with radiology

In any child who has not achieved menarche, further follow up will be required for a cyst of any size.

Reference:
BritSPAG: Guideline for the management of ovarian cysts in children and adolescents, June 2017

38. **M** Provoked vulvodynia is the most likely diagnosis in light of normal examination and localized, provoked tenderness.

39. **F** Lichen sclerosus is the most likely cause with pale, white skin appearance and complete loss of architecture.

40. **E** Erosive lichen planus is the most likely diagnosis with the vulvo-vaginal-gingival triad of symptoms found.

Reference:
BASHH. UK National Guideline on the Management of Vulval Conditions. February 2014.

41. **L** Where the patient has not responded to conservative measures (including drug therapy) and has declined/or is unsuitable for botulinum toxin treatment then percutaneous sacral nerve stimulation can be considered after MDT review.

Reference:
NICE guideline CG171: Urinary incontinence in women; September 2013, last updated 2015.

42. **I** Mirabegron is the best option for treatment given her age and frailty. NICE guidelines suggest avoidance of anti-cholinergics in frail, older patients.

References:
NICE guideline TA290: Mirabegron for treating symptoms of overactive bladder; June 2013.

NICE guideline CG171: Urinary incontinence in women; September 2013, last updated November 2015.

43. **C** Desmopressin can be offered to women with urge incontinence or OAB where nocturia is a troublesome symptom. Caution must be used in women with cystic fibrosis and avoid in those over 65 years with cardiovascular disease or hypertension.

Reference:
NICE guideline CG171: Urinary incontinence in women; September 2013, last updated November 2015

44. D Duloxetine should not be offered routinely as a second line treatment but can be used where patients have a contraindication/decline surgical management.

Reference:
NICE guideline CG171 : Urinary incontinence in women; September 2013, last updated November 2015.

45. F Kallman's syndrome

46. L Turner's syndrome.

	MRKH	CAIS	SWYER	TURNER
Chromosomes	46 XX	46XY	46XY	45XO
Vagina	Dimple	Blind ending	Yes	Yes
Uterus	No	No	Yes	Yes
Axillary hair	Yes	Yes	No	No
Breasts	Yes	No	No	No
Gonads	Yes	Streak	Streak	Yes

Reference:
Paediatric and Adolescent Gynaecology for the MRCOG and Beyond, 2nd edition, August 2008

47. O A continuous or cyclical (day 15-28) low dose SSRI would be indicated in this case where mood disorder is the primary feature and her menorrhagia has greatly improved with tranexamic acid. CBT should also be an option if it is available in her area.

48. K When treating women with severe PMS; hysterectomy and bilateral oophorectomy can be considered when medical management has failed, long-term GnRH analogue treatment is required or other gynaecological conditions indicate surgery. When treating women with PMS, surgery should not be contemplated without preoperative use of GnRH analogues as a test of cure and to ensure that HRT is tolerated.

49. F GnRH analogues may be used for 3 months for a definitive diagnosis if the completed symptom diary alone is inconclusive.

50. B When treating women with PMS, emerging data suggest use of the contraceptive pill continuously rather than cyclically. When treating women with PMS, drospirenone-containing COCs may represent effective treatment and should be considered as a first-line pharmaceutical intervention. CBT should be considered routinely as a treatment option.

Reference:
RCOG Green-Top Guideline No. 48: Management of Premenstrual syndrome, November 2016.

Anti-D Administration Checklist

Always confirm
- the woman's identity
- that the woman is RhD Negative using the latest laboratory report
- that the woman does not have immune anti-D using the latest laboratory report
- that informed consent for administration of anti-D Ig is recorded in notes

Potentially Sensitising Events (PSEs) during pregnancy

Gestation LESS than 12 weeks	
Vaginal bleeding associated with severe pain	Administer at least **250 IU** anti-D Ig within **72 hours** of event. Confirm product / dose / expiry and patient ID pre administration
ERPC / Instrumentation of uterus	
Medical or surgical termination of pregnancy	
Ectopic / Molar Pregnancy	

Gestation 12 to 20 weeks	
For any Potentially Sensitising Event (PSE)	Administer at least **250 IU** anti-D Ig within **72 hours** of event. Confirm product / dose / expiry and patient ID pre administration

Gestation 20 weeks to term	
For any Potentially Sensitising Event (PSE) (**Irrespective** of whether RAADP has been given)	Request a Kleihauer Test (FMH Test) and immediately administer at least **500 IU** anti-D Ig within **72 hours** of event. Confirm product / dose / expiry and patient ID pre administration
Does the Kleihauer / FMH test indicate that further anti-D Ig is required ?	Administer more anti-D Ig following discussion with laboratory

For continuous vaginal bleeding at least 500iu anti-D Ig should be administered at a minimum of 6-weekly intervals, irrespective of the presence of detectable anti-D, and a Kleihauer Test requested every two weeks in case more anti-D is needed

Routine Antenatal Anti-D Prophylaxis (RAADP)

For Routine Antenatal Anti-D Prophylaxis (**Irrespective** of whether anti-D Ig already given for PSE)	Take a blood sample to confirm group & check antibody screen – do not wait for results before administering anti-D Ig
	Administer **1500 IU** anti-D Ig at **28 – 30** weeks
	OR
	Administer at least **500 IU** anti-D Ig at **28** weeks and then administer at least **500 IU** anti-D at **34** weeks
	Confirm product / dose / expiry and patient ID pre administration

At Delivery (or on diagnosis of Intra Uterine Death >20 weeks)

Is the baby's group confirmed as RhD positive ? OR Are cord samples not available ?	Request a Kleihauer Test (FMH Test)
	Administer at least **500 IU** anti-D Ig within **72 hours** of delivery. Confirm product / dose / expiry and patient ID pre administration
Does the Kleihauer / FMH test indicate that further anti-D Ig is required ?	Administer more anti-D following discussion with laboratory

Obstetric paper 2 - Answers

1.H Women with a history of second-trimester miscarriage and suspected cervical weakness who have not undergone a history-indicated cerclage may be offered serial cervical sonographic surveillance. In this case with a cervical excision depth of 17mm, the meta-analysis by Kyrgiou et al. (2006) reported that excisional treatment which exceeded 10mm in length increased prematurity.

References:
Green-Top Guideline No 17: The investigation and treatment of couples with recurrent first trimester and second trimester miscarriage; April 2011.

Scientific Impact Paper No. 21: Reproductive outcomes after local treatment for pre-invasive cervical disease, July 2016.

Kyrgiou M, Koliopoulos G, Martin-Hirsch P, Arbyn M, Prendiville W, Paraskevaidis E. Obstetric outcomes after conservative treatment for intraepithelial or early invasive cervical lesions: systematic review and meta-analysis. Lancet 2006;367:489–98.

2.H In women with a singleton pregnancy and a history of one second-trimester miscarriage attributable to cervical factors, an ultrasound-indicated cerclage should be offered if a cervical length of 25 mm or less is detected by transvaginal scan before 24 weeks of gestation.

Reference:
Green-Top Guideline No 17: The investigation and treatment of couples with recurrent first trimester and second trimester miscarriage; April 2011.

3. J Offer prophylactic vaginal progesterone to women with no history of spontaneous preterm birth or mid-trimester loss in whom a transvaginal ultrasound scan has been carried out between 16+0 and 24+0 weeks of pregnancy that reveals a cervical length of less than 25 mm.

Reference:
NICE Guideline No 25: Preterm labour and birth, November 2015.

4. H Consider prophylactic cervical cerclage for women in whom a transvaginal ultrasound scan has been carried out between 16+0 and 24+0 weeks of pregnancy that reveals a cervical length of less than 25 mm and who have either:

- preterm pre-labour rupture of membranes (P-PROM) in a previous pregnancy
- a history of cervical trauma.

Reference:
As above

5. O Antenatal risk factors for this lady: BMI 45, PE after surgery. Her VTE risk score is 4 therefore she needs 60mg enoxaparin once daily from 12 weeks gestation until at least 6 weeks postnatal.

6. J Antenatal risk factors for this lady: antithrombin deficiency and previous DVTs/PE. This lady has already had DVTs/PE in the past on the background of a thrombophilia hence she will need both antenatal and postnatal prophylaxis until she can be switched back to warfarin. The correct dose given her weight is 5000iu dalteparin once daily.

Obstetric paper 2 – Answers

7. A Antenatal risk factors for this lady: IVDU and heterozygous factor V Leiden. Her VTE risk score is 4 hence she needs early antenatal and 6 weeks postnatal thromboprophylaxis. Given her low weight she would require dalteparin 2500iu once daily.

8. P Antenatal risk factors for this lady: BMI 38, gross varicose veins, early PET. Antenatally her VTE risk score is 3 hence prophylaxis should be offered from 28 weeks and should continue postnatally for 6 weeks as her post-natal risk score will be at least 4 (P3, BMI 38, varicose veins, PET). Given her weight, a dose of 60mg enoxaparin once daily is required.

References: (see RCOG guideline summary tables on pages 115 to 118)

RCOG Green-top Guideline No 37a: Reducing the risk of venous thromboembolism during pregnancy and the puerperium, April 2015

RCOG Green-top Guideline No 37b: Thromboembolic disease in pregnancy and the puerperium; acute management, April 2015

9. C Once the scapula is visible, the arms can be hooked down by inserting a finger in the elbow and flexing the arms across the chest or, if nuchal, Lovset's manoeuvre is advised. Delivery is achieved either with the Mauriceau-Smellie-Veit manoeuvre or with forceps. Suprapubic pressure will aid flexion if there is delay due to an extended neck. Delivery using the Burns-Marshall technique is not advised due to concern of overextension of the foetal neck.

10.O Women near or in active second stage of labour should not be routinely offered Caesarean section. Where time and circumstances permit, the position of the foetal neck and legs, and the foetal weight should be estimated using ultrasound, and the woman counselled as with planned vaginal breech birth.

Reference:
RCOG Green-Top Guideline No. 20b: Management of breech presentation; March 2017

11.J In the event of continual uterine bleeding which is clinically judged to represent the same sensitising event, with no features suggestive of a new presentation or a significant change in the pattern or severity of bleeding, such as the presence of abdominal pain or another clinical presentation, a minimum dose of 500 IU anti-D Ig should be given at six weekly intervals. In the event of further intermittent uterine bleeding, estimation of FMH should be carried out at two weekly intervals. In this situation non-invasive foetal RHD typing using maternal plasma could be considered to reduce hospital attendance, blood sampling and avoid repeated administration of doses of anti-D, balanced against the small risk of false negativity of foetal D typing by this technique.

12.H If there is an intrauterine death (IUD) no foetal sample can be obtained from the umbilical cord so prophylactic anti-D Ig should be administered to D-negative, previously non-sensitised women. A minimum of 500 IU of anti-D Ig should be administered within 72 hours following the diagnosis of IUD. Maternal samples should be tested for FMH and additional dose(s) given as guided by FMH tests. It should be noted that the diagnosis of IUD is the sensitising event rather than delivery and hence anti-D Ig should be administered within 72 hours of diagnosis.

Reference:
BCSH Guideline for the use of anti-D immunoglobulin for the prevention of haemolytic disease of the foetus and newborn, 2014

13.G There is an increased risk of pulmonary embolism among women with SCD. In women presenting with acute hypoxia, there should be a low threshold for considering PE. In this situation, therapeutic low-molecular-weight heparin should be commenced until the lady has been reviewed by senior staff and definitive investigations have been undertaken.

14.D ACS is characterised by fever and/or respiratory symptoms combined with a new pulmonary infiltrate found on CXR. Early recognition of ACS is key. Treatment is with intravenous antibiotics, oxygen, analgesia and blood transfusion, as in non-pregnant women. Top-up blood transfusion may be required if the haemoglobin is falling, and certainly if the haemoglobin is less than 6.5 g/dl, but in severe hypoxia, and if the haemoglobin level is maintained, exchange transfusion will be required. If ACS is suspected, the woman should be reviewed urgently by the haematology team to advise on transfusion. If the woman has hypoxia, she should be reviewed by the critical care team and ventilatory support may be required.

References:
RCOG Green Top Guideline No. 61: Management of sickle cell disease in pregnancy, July 2011.

British Society for Haematology. Management of acute chest syndrome in sickle cell disease. March 2015.

15. E

16. F

17. K

Reference:
NICE Guideline: Hypertension in pregnancy: Diagnosis and management; January 2011

18.C An anti-c level of > 7.5 iu/ml but < 20 iu/ml correlates with a moderate risk of HDFN, whereas an anti-c level of > 20 iu/ml correlates with a high risk of HDFN. Referral for a foetal medicine opinion should therefore be made once anti-c levels are > 7.5 iu/ml. Referral to a foetal medicine specialist for consideration of invasive treatment should take place if the MCA PSV rises above 1.5 MoM or if there are other signs of foetal anaemia. MCA PSV monitoring is predictive of moderate or severe foetal anaemia with 100% sensitivity and a false positive rate of 12%. If monitoring of the MCA indicates anaemia (MCA PSV > 1.5 MoM), foetal blood sampling (FBS) and potential IUT are indicated.

19.I Where clinically significant maternal red cell antibodies are detected, the paternal phenotype can be ascertained by serology. However with the rhesus D (RhD) antigen specifically, in an antigen-positive father, while a likely phenotype can be deduced, genotyping is required to determine whether he is homozygous or heterozygous for the RHD gene. If the father is homozygous for the red cell antigen then all pregnancies are potentially at risk. Genotyping can be undertaken from 16 weeks gestation for all except K antigen.

20.J Where clinically significant maternal red cell antibodies are detected, the paternal phenotype can be ascertained by serology. However if the father is homozygous for the red cell antigen then all pregnancies are potentially at risk. Genotyping can be undertaken from 20 weeks gestation for K antigen as there is a higher risk of a false-negative result if performed earlier in pregnancy.

Reference:
RCOG Green-Top Guideline No. 65: The management of women with red cell antibodies during pregnancy; May 2014

Obstetric paper 2 – Answers

21. H Antenatal treatment is not recommended for GBS cultured from a vaginal or rectal swab. Where GBS carriage is detected incidentally or by intentional testing, women should be offered IAP.

22. F IAP is recommended for women in confirmed preterm labour.

23. F Birth in a pool is not contraindicated if the woman is a known GBS carrier provided she is offered appropriate IAP.

24. N How should known or unknown GBS carrier status be managed in women with preterm prelabour rupture of membranes? For those with evidence of colonisation in the current pregnancy or in previous pregnancies, the perinatal risks associated with preterm delivery at less than 34+0 weeks of gestation are likely to outweigh the risk of perinatal infection. For those at more than 34+0 weeks of gestation it may be beneficial to expedite delivery if a woman is a known GBS carrier.

25. I Provided a woman has not had severe allergy to penicillin, a cephalosporin should be used. If there is any evidence of severe allergy to penicillin, vancomycin should be used.

Reference:
RCOG Guideline No. 36: Prevention of early onset neonatal group B streptococcal disease, September 2017

26. E When repairing the vaginal mucosa a rapidly absorbable, undyed, braided suture such as a 2-0 polyglactin should be used.

Reference:
Kettle T et al, June 2010. Absorbable suture materials for primary repair of episiotomy and second degree tears. Cochrane Database of Systematic Reviews.

27.H Extra-corporeal suturing using a 2-0 polyglactin (vicryl) suture on a small curved needle should be considered.

28.I This is a biological suture synthesised from the collagen of bovine intestines. Its use was discontinued in Europe following the BSE scare in the 1980s.

29. L Monocryl is a monofilament suture which maintains its tensile strength for up to 4 weeks and is not completely absorbed for up to 120 days.

Reference:
Raghavan R, Arya P, Arya P, China S. Abdominal incisions and sutures in obstetrics and gynaecology. The Obstetrician & Gynaecologist 2014;16:13–18.

30.L The optimal management of this patient would be for administration of anti-D in keeping with current guidelines; however without patient consent no treatment can be given. Provided she undergoes sterilization as intended she would be very unlikely to have a further pregnancy and risk of HDN.

31.J Where intra-operative cell salvage (ICS) is used during Caesarean section in D negative, non-sensitised women and where cord blood group is confirmed as D positive (or unknown), a minimum dose of 1500 IU anti-D Ig should be administered following the re-infusion of salvaged red cells. A maternal blood sample should be taken for estimation of FMH 30–45 minutes after reinfusion, in case more anti-D Ig is indicated. The clinician should inform the transfusion laboratory if ICS has been used, to ensure that the correct dose of anti-D Ig is issued.

Obstetric paper 2 – Answers

32. A Whenever possible, D negative platelets should be transfused to D negative girls or women of child bearing potential who need a platelet transfusion. Occasionally, if the appropriate product is not available or its availability would cause an unacceptable delay, it may be necessary to transfuse D positive platelets. In these circumstances, prophylaxis against possible sensitisation to the D antigen by red cells contaminating the platelet product should be given. A dose of 250 IU anti-D immunoglobulin should be sufficient to cover up to five adult therapeutic doses of D positive platelets given within a 6-week period. In severely thrombocytopenic patients with platelet count of ≤30 × 10 9/L, anti-D Ig should be given subcutaneously, or IV if a preparation suitable or IV route is available, to avoid the risk of IM bleed following IM injection.

Reference:
BCSH guideline for the use of anti-D immunoglobulin for the prevention of haemolytic disease of the foetus and newborn,
Transfusion Medicine, 2014, 24,8–20.

See the checklist on page 136

33.L 2:1000 risk.

34.K 1:1000 risk.

35.J 0.5:1000 risk.

Reference:
RCOG Green Top Guideline nr 20b: Management of breech presentation; March 2017

36. K Due to lack of safety data, all chelation therapy should be regarded as potentially teratogenic in the first trimester. Desferrioxamine is the only chelation agent with a body of evidence for use in the second and third trimester. The optimisation of iron burden is therefore critical as the ongoing iron accumulation from transfusions (in the absence of chelation) may expose the pregnant woman to a high risk of new complications related to iron overload, particularly diabetes and cardiomyopathy. Cardiac assessment is important to determine cardiac function and possible further iron chelation as well as planning for labour. Women with myocardial iron loading should undergo regular cardiology review with careful monitoring of ejection fraction during the pregnancy as signs of cardiac decompensation are the primary indications for intervention with chelation therapy. Those women at highest risk of cardiac decompensation should commence low-dose subcutaneous desferrioxamine (20 mg/kg/day) on a minimum of 4–5 days a week under joint haematology and cardiology guidance from 20–24 weeks of gestation.

37. K If liver iron exceeds 15 mg/g (dw) prior to conception, the risk of myocardial iron loading increases, so iron chelation with low-dose desferrioxamine should be commenced between 20 and 28 weeks under guidance from the haemoglobinopathy team.

Reference:
RCOG Green-top Guideline No. 66: Management of beta thalassaemia in pregnancy, March 2014.

Obstetric paper 2 – Answers

38. D For the purposes of the MBRRACE-UK report, extended perinatal death refers to all stillbirths and neonatal deaths.

39. E Maternal death.

40. I Maternal mortality ratio.

References:
MBRRACE-UK perinatal mortality surveillance report - UK perinatal deaths for 2015 Births: Definitions page iii.

The WHO application of ICD-10 to deaths during pregnancy, childbirth and puerperium: ICD MM, WHO 2012.

International statistical classification of diseases and related health problems. 10th revised edition 2010.

41. C 1:10

42. I 3-6:1000

43. F 9:100.

References:
Caesarean section for placenta praevia, Consent advice no.12, December 2010

Operative vaginal delivery, Consent advice no.11, July 2010

Repair of third and fourth degree tears following childbirth, Consent advice no.9, June 2010

44. D Women who breastfeed should be advised not to breastfeed and to express and discard milk for a week after they have taken UPA-EC

45. I Women who are breastfeeding should wait until 6 weeks after childbirth before initiating a CHC method.

46. H IUC can be safely inserted immediately after birth (within 10 minutes of delivery of the placenta) or within the first 48 hours after uncomplicated Caesarean section or vaginal birth. After 48 hours, insertion should be delayed until 28 days after childbirth.

47. O Women should be advised that IMP can be safely initiated at the time of mifepristone administration.

Reference:
FSRH Guideline: Contraception after pregnancy, January 2017.

Obstetric paper 2 – Answers

48. J The death of a woman from direct or indirect obstetric causes, more than 42 days, but less than one year after the end of pregnancy.

49. K Direct obstetric deaths are those resulting from obstetric complications of the pregnancy state (pregnancy, labour and the puerperium), from interventions, omissions, incorrect treatment, or from a chain of events resulting from any of the above.

50. N Coincidental deaths that occur during pregnancy, childbirth and puerperium are not considered as maternal deaths as such.

References: (see summary table on page 119)
MBRRACE-UK perinatal mortality surveillance report - UK perinatal deaths for 2015 births: Definitions page iii.

The WHO application of ICD-10 to deaths during pregnancy, childbirth and puerperium: ICD MM, WHO 2012.

International statistical classification of diseases and related health problems. 10th revised edition 2010.